LEGISLATION TO REAUTHORIZE THE NATIONAL INSTITUTES OF HEALTH

HEARING

BEFORE THE

COMMITTEE ON ENERGY AND COMMERCE

HOUSE OF REPRESENTATIVES

ONE HUNDRED NINTH CONGRESS

FIRST SESSION

JULY 19, 2005

Serial No. 109–40

Printed for the use of the Committee on Energy and Commerce

Available via the World Wide Web: http://www.access.gpo.gov/congress/house

U.S. GOVERNMENT PRINTING OFFICE

22–987PDF

WASHINGTON : 2005

CONTENTS

Page

Testimony of:
    Zerhouni, Elias A., Director, National Institutes of Health 10
Additional material submitted for the record:
    Zerhouni, Elias A., Director, National Institutes of Health, response for
      the record 65

(III)

LEGISLATION TO REAUTHORIZE THE NATIONAL INSTITUTES OF HEALTH

TUESDAY, JULY 19, 2005

House of Representatives,
Committee on Energy and Commerce,
Washington, DC.

The committee met, pursuant to notice, at 2 p.m., in room 2318 of the Rayburn House Office Building, Hon. Nathan Deal (acting chairman) presiding.

Members present: Representatives Barton, Bilirakis, Deal, Wilson, Buyer, Pitts, Walden, Ferguson, Rogers, Myrick, Murphy, Burgess, Blackburn, Waxman, Markey, Towns, Brown, Rush, Eshoo, Stupak, Engel, Wynn, Green, DeGette, Capps, Allen, Solis, Inslee, and Baldwin.

Staff present: Chuck Clapton, chief health counsel; Cheryl Jaeger, majority professional staff; Eugenia Edwards, legislative clerk; Brandon Clark, health policy coordinator; John Ford, minority counsel; and Voncille Hines, minority research assistant.

Mr. Deal. I call this hearing to order. I need to explain to our witness, and to the rest of the committee that our chairman and some of our members of this committee are engaged in the Energy Conference, and therefore, they may come in, and they may have to leave. So—and the fact that they are meeting right now—we decided to proceed on with this hearing today, and I believe we have enough to proceed.

I recognize myself for a very brief opening statement. First of all, I want to welcome Dr. Zerhouni to this hearing, and it is a hearing in our continuing effort to reauthorize the National Institutes of Health, and we appreciate you for joining us again, as you have in the past. This is an area of jurisdiction that is important to this committee, and many of you are aware that this is actually the eleventh hearing we have had on NIH in the last 2½ years, and all of us are hopeful that the result of those hearings and the work of our staffs will allow us to achieve the very important function of reauthorizing NIH.

We have been working on the issue of reauthorization of NIH for longer than many people on this committee have actually been in— serving in Congress, and some of us are of the opinion that now is the time to finalize that issue, and we are hopeful of doing that in the very near future. One of the issues that is important, I think, to all of us on this committee, regardless of our party affiliation, is the fact that in the absence of reauthorizing NIH, this committee basically cedes its jurisdiction to another committee, namely, the Appropriations Committee, and we believe that it is appropriate for us to reclaim that issue of jurisdiction, and this effort to reauthorize will do that.

Times have changed, and certainly, as times change, the necessity of looking at organizations such as NIH, and whether or not it, too, should change is indeed appropriate. Dr. Zerhouni, again, we welcome your attendance today, and look forward to hearing your testimony and working with you as we proceed with NIH reauthorization.

I am now pleased to recognize my ranking member of our subcommittee, but I presume standing in also for the full committee, Mr. Brown of Ohio.

[The prepared statement of Hon. Nathan Deal follows:]

PREPARED STATEMENT OF HON. NATHAN DEAL, CHAIRMAN, SUBCOMMITTEE ON HEALTH

Thank you, Mr. Chairman.

I want to start off by welcoming Dr. Zerhouni to this hearing on our efforts to reauthorize the National Institutes of Health. We appreciate your joining us again this afternoon to talk about one of the most important priorities under the jurisdiction of this Committee.

As you are well aware, this will be the Energy and Commerce Committee's *eleventh* hearing on the NIH in last two and a half years, and we are hopeful we can all continue to work together to achieve some much-needed improvements to this vital component of our federal government.

As many of you know, we have been working on reauthorizing the NIH longer than most of the Members of this Committee have been serving in Congress, and it is *well past* time for this Committee to get something done.

Indeed, Mr. Chairman, it is time for Authorizers to be Authorizers again, and I applaud you for your leadership on this very important issue.

Times change and organizations must adapt to this change. We must modernize the organizational structure of the NIH so that we can advance scientific discovery for the benefit of all mankind.

Again, Dr. Zerhouni we appreciate your attendance and expertise, and we look forward to working with you as we strive to improve one of the most important agencies in our government.

Mr. BROWN. Thank you, Mr. Chairman, and thank you, Dr. Zerhouni, as always, for joining us with your wisdom and your knowledge. It is our responsibility to ensure that agencies under our jurisdiction have the resources and statutory authority they need to advance the public good. NIH represents half the discretionary budget at HHS, and the chairman has rightly assigned a high priority to its reauthorization.

As we know, NIH is a complex agency. Its work affects the lives of millions of Americans. I want to make it clear that passing a consensus, a consensus bill, requires that all parties have the necessary time to contribute their ideas, perspective, and insight into the final product, and I would reiterate, have the necessary time to contribute these ideas and perspective.

Well, this committee has had numerous hearings on NIH. The devil, of course, is in the details. Members of Congress and stakeholder groups have had less than a week to review legislation that translates general concepts into concrete operational changes in a very complicated structure, as I have seen from both committee hearings and individual personal conversations with Dr. Zerhouni. We need time to make sure the bill does what we think it does, and that those changes are beneficial. However, given the right timeframe, and with the right input from inside Congress and outside Congress, I am confident we can pass a bill that represents true progress for NIH and for all of the American public.

Thank you.

Mr. DEAL. Thank the gentleman. Does anyone else wish to make an opening statement?

Mr. BILIRAKIS. Just a very brief one.

Mr. DEAL. Mr. Bilirakis.

Mr. BILIRAKIS. Just a very brief one, Mr. Chairman.

I am one of those people who will probably have to be called upon at a moment's notice to go downstairs for a vote on the conference, but I did want to join you and the others in welcoming Dr. Zerhouni here, and to thank you for your part in the preparation of this legislation.

We must reauthorize NIH. I think we all agree to that, to increase transparency and accountability at the agency, and to ensure that it is operating as effectively and efficiently as possible. And I would also like to say, and really emphasize, Mr. Chairman, that we must make certain that any changes that we make to NIH will not harm its various institutes. I am always concerned about the unintended consequences of our acts. Haste sometimes makes waste. We are all—have our minds made up that we are going to reauthorize this time around. We are working with the minority, which is just great in that regard, but let us make sure that we are concerned that our—whatever we do do, and whatever changes we do make will not cause more harm than good.

So having said that, Mr. Chairman, I would yield back, and thank you.

Mr. DEAL. Thank the gentleman. Anyone else. Mr. Rush?

Mr. RUSH. Thank you, Mr. Chairman. Mr. Chairman, I also want to thank you for holding this hearing, and I will be brief, since my time in short, and we want to really get to hear Dr. Zerhouni.

Mr. Chairman, I truly appreciate your leadership in this committee reasserting its jurisdiction over the National Institutes of Health. For too long, the appropriators have had way too much authority over NIH, and it is time that this committee put an end to that reign. With all due respect to that other committee, we are the committee of expertise, and it serves this Congress, the NIH, and the American people well when we utilize that expertise.

Having that said, I have two key issues that I would like to— the draft legislation before us to address. First, I remain concerned that the issue of racial disparities, an old, shameful problem that has not gone away, and Dr. Zerhouni, in his statement, agrees with this point, that the issue of racial disparities is not adequately addressed by this bill. We need stronger mandates for our premier medical research institute to aggressively address an inexcusable and unconstitutional problem in our country here. Specifically, I want to hear what NIH can do to include more people of color and women in clinical trials, both as researchers themselves, and as subjects in the private sector.

Second, I am concerned that medical research in this country is not adequately incorporating children in their research and medical deliberations. I believe that NIH needs to consider the pros and cons of including children in clinical trials, and use its leverage and Federal dollars accordingly.

As always, I welcome the Director to this hearing, and I look forward to his testimony. And Mr. Chairman, I look forward to working with you and the rest of the members of this committee, so that we can come up with a truly bipartisan, cooperative, and deliberative piece of legislation that reauthorizes the National Institutes of Health.

I yield back the balance of my time.

Mr. DEAL. Thank the gentleman. I recognize Ms. Wilson for an opening statement.

Ms. WILSON. Thank you, Mr. Chairman, and thank you for holding this hearing.

I think there are some concepts in this draft legislation that are worth supporting, certainly in prioritizing the research in the most promising areas, and allowing greater flexibility to manage research roadmaps across the various institutes of the National Institutes of Health, and second, to give the Director authority over a certain percentage of funding to direct particular research—and there is a precedent in this area, with the Department of Energy Laboratories, where a certain percentage is set aside for lab-directed research and development, to put money toward the most promising research.

There are a couple of areas I think we need to be attentive to. One is that this legislation tries to move forward on establishing an electronic data base of research projects, which is very helpful to those who are looking for clinical trials, and information about research ongoing. I think we need to make sure that that data base is publicly available, not just to people who are researchers or medical doctors, but accessible to the public, who are paying for this research, that it is searchable, and it really does enhance access to clinical trials.

The second area where I have some concerns has to do with public/private coordination or collaboration. The legislation does anticipate some partnership in high risk and high reward areas of research, but I wonder whether we should limit those collaborative mechanisms to just the high risk research, and whether we should expand those mechanisms and encouragement to include basic research, because there is a lot more research that is done outside of the NIH than is done inside of the NIH, and collaboration and coordination could, I think, help both.

And with those two caveats, I look forward to the testimony today. Thank you, Mr. Chairman.

Mr. DEAL. Thank the gentlelady. Mr. Waxman, do you have an opening statement?

Mr. WAXMAN. Yes, Mr. Chairman.

The National Institutes of Health is, without doubt, one of the premiere agencies in the Federal Government. It is widely respected throughout the world. It is an agency with a mission critical to the Nation's health; and it is an agency that few would dispute is working well.

Can it do better? Of course. Where it can be strengthened, we want to do that. All of us want to provide the necessary tools to enhance its ability to perform its mission. But this is not an agency which is broken. The changes we make to improve it must be thoughtful and measured, and we must be certain that we are not unintentionally taking actions which reduce the very features that have made it strong.

Our goal, as authorizers of this institution, should not be to restrict the resources the agency receives, but to provide fully for its support and growth now and into the future. Our goal should be to maintain and defend the peer review process which is at the heart of its strength, and to give the Institutes the tools to stay at the forefront of medical research.

I look forward to hearing from Dr. Zerhouni today, and from any other persons and institutions who support and benefit from the work of this agency. And I hope and trust this committee will move forward with caution and care and deliberation.

Thank you.

Mr. DEAL. Thank the gentleman. Anyone on this side have—Dr. Burgess, recognized for an opening statement.

Mr. BURGESS. Thank you, Mr. Chairman, and I, too, appreciate your holding this hearing today, and I know that this reauthorization is one of your highest priorities, and I think we can see the fruits of your labor before us today, and of course, welcome again the Director of the NIH, Dr. Zerhouni, and I am looking forward to his comments on the draft bill.

On my review, I think the draft does strike a balance of achievable reforms. Granting the Director greater budgetary authority will go a long way in redirecting research priorities at the NIH. With additional oversight and authority, the NIH director can plan, in a more strategic manner, and respond to emergencies as they occur.

I have visited the NIH. I have visited with the Director, and you really get a sense of how precious that organization is to this country. In fact, it is my visit to the NIH that is one of the few things of the last 2½ years that have really made me optimistic about the future of this country that we are leaving to our children and grandchildren.

The research conducted by the NIH is truly groundbreaking, whether it is additional treatment for cancer or a greater understanding of the human genome, the NIH has a proven record of innovation. Improvements can be made in its managerial structure, and that is, in fact, how we will improve the quality of research conducted at NIH and the health of all Americans.

Thank you, Mr. Chairman. I will yield back.

Mr. DEAL. Thank the gentleman. Anyone else? Mr. Engel.

Mr. ENGEL. Thank you, Mr. Chairman. At the outset, I would like to say that I like sitting on this side of the committee. I want to thank you for——

Mr. DEAL. You have to act accordingly.

Mr. ENGEL. I want to thank you for convening this hearing today. I am very pleased to welcome Dr. Zerhouni back for his seventh appearance before our committee.

It is always good to see you, Doctor. It is disappointing, though, that none of the stakeholders that will be affected by the proposed restructuring of the NIH were invited to give their reaction to these proposals. I certainly support initiatives to improve coordination and increase transparency among the NIH institutes and centers. The proposed concentration of budget, management, and grant making authority in the office of the NIH, though, may go further than necessary to achieve these goals.

I am concerned that the discussion draft establishes four specific authorizations of appropriations line items, which may dramatically impact the ability of the constituencies of the 27 research institutes and centers from having a place at the table in the appropriations process. I am not certain that authorizing the virtual elimination of these important relationships is the best policy proposal.

I appreciate the commitment of the chairman to open and amend the proposed legislation based on feedback from members of this committee and the many stakeholders who work with and benefit from NIH research. As we move forward, it is my sincere hope that we can pass legislation that strengthens the management of the NIH without sacrificing the voices of these important groups.

I thank you, and I yield back.

Mr. DEAL. Thank the gentleman. Mr. Ferguson.

Mr. FERGUSON. Does that mean we have to act accordingly on this side, Mr. Chairman?

Mr. DEAL. You are excused.

Mr. FERGUSON. Thank you, Mr. Chairman. I certainly thank Dr. Zerhouni for being here again with us today, and certainly looking forward to the reauthorization process.

The NIH is a place where groundbreaking research occurs daily, research that might lead to a cure for many of the diseases that affect people throughout our world. Recently, Congress has set out on an ambitious path to increase funding for NIH, and we have seen the budget double in the last number of years. We have not seen NIH reauthorized in 12 years, since 1993, and recent hearings have pointed to a need for interagency cooperation and coordination to help maximize the resources of the Institutes.

We must give the Director the ability to manage the NIH portfolio to focus on research that yields results, cures to diseases that are within reach. In the January 2004 edition of Health Affairs, Dr. Zerhouni said: "We need to be able to plan across NIH. We need some funds in common. If you have 27 fingers out there with no palm, you don't have a hand."

I look forward to this hearing, to hear Dr. Zerhouni's impressions of the hand that you have been dealt, and what we can do to give you the upper hand as we go through the reauthorization process, and as we try to enable NIH to find the cures to diseases which affect so many people throughout the world.

Thank you, Mr. Chairman. I yield back.

Mr. DEAL. Oh, well, at least we don't have a paradox today. Recognize Ms. DeGette.

Ms. DEGETTE. Thank you, Mr. Chairman, and I would like to add my welcome to Dr. Zerhouni.

The last time we authorized the NIH was 12 years ago in the House, and when you think about the status of medical research 12 years ago, you really realize why reauthorization of this important agency is well overdue. The nature of medical research and, frankly, the integration of research that we are seeing among the 27 Institutes has grown dramatically in the last 12 years.

I agree with Mr. Waxman. The system is not broken, and that is why it is such a pleasure to be reauthorizing the agency at this juncture. But I think it is important that we discuss what the balance is between the 27 fingers and the palm of the agency, and we really try to figure out how we can keep the autonomy and the important research that is happening among those 27 agencies, but at the same time, use the Director's Office to ensure that cross-fertilization happens in the important way that it can, because that is the only way that we will really see medical research advance in the 21st Century.

Thank you, Mr. Chairman.

Mr. DEAL. Thank the gentlelady. Anyone else on this side have an opening statement? If not, anyone on the top row here? Yes. Mr. Stupak.

Mr. STUPAK. Thank you, Mr. Chairman. Dr. Zerhouni, thanks for coming here today. I look forward to your comments.

Since I have 1 minute, I am going to focus on one area of this draft legislation that I find troubling. The draft strikes a section of the Public Health Service Act that authorizes pediatric drug studies at NIH. This Section, 409(i)(d), was added in 201 as part of the Best Pharmaceuticals for Children Act. The BPCA reauthorized a law that gave drug companies patent extensions in exchange for testing the drugs on children. The incentive doesn't work if the drug has no patent protection left, therefore Congress created a research fund within NIH to study drugs that are off patent.

It is one of only a few provisions in law that actually mandates FDA and NIH to work together on drug safety. This draft would strike that provision. The sad fact is that Congress has never funded this provision, but it does not mean it is not important. It is more important than ever. Off-label use by children of drugs approved and labeled only for adults is rampant. The FDA has no power to restrict off-label use, and the list of drugs that need to be studied continues to grow. If the FDA cannot or will not enforce drug companies to do these studies, then at the very least, we should not eliminate a safeguard that gives parents some assurance that their children's drugs will be tested for safety and efficacy.

I look forward to working with this committee on this issue, and will be submitting additional questions to the record. Thank you, Mr. Chairman.

Mr. DEAL. I thank the gentleman. I might tell him that due note has been made of your concerns, and will be addressed in the next draft.

Mr. Allen.

Mr. ALLEN. Thank you, Mr. Chairman. Welcome, Dr. Zerhouni. I hope you enjoyed your brief visit to Maine, and I want to thank you for your leadership at NIH.

I just wanted to mention several concerns about this draft. First, the committee needs adequate time to consider this legislation, and to obtain input from stakeholders. Second, a question. To what degree should the Director have the authority to add, remove, and transfer Institute responsibilities without ensuring a transparent public process? I do worry that the concentration of so much power in the office of the Director could result, could, in ideological and political considerations trumping good science.

Third, this draft legislation appears to create an arbitrary ceiling of Federal investment in biomedical research. Establishing a ceiling would seem to directly contradict Congressional success in doubling the NIH research budget, and imposing a ceiling could also hamper the agency's ability to deal with new public health threats. We just passed an appropriations bill with the smallest increase for NIH in 36 years, so at least now, the budget is growing slower than the costs of inflation and new research.

Finally, I believe that legislation to reauthorize the NIH should address the violations of NIH scientists engaging in outside consulting agreements with pharmaceutical companies, and I want to commend Chairman Barton and Ranking Member Dingell for their leadership on this particular issue.

I look forward to hearing from you, and with that, Mr. Chairman, I yield back.

Mr. DEAL. I thank the gentleman. Ms. Solis.

Ms. SOLIS. Thank you, Mr. Chairman, and welcome, Dr. Elias Zerhouni. I am very interested in hearing what your testimony will reveal to us today.

But one of the concerns I have is, I happen to represent a very diverse district in Southern California, where we are finding that access to health care, as you know, is a crisis—it is in a crisis stage for many of the constituents I represent. But more importantly, the diverse communities, not only in Southern California, but across the country, we increasingly see that there is a lack of research being done in these different racial and ethnic minority communities. We are trying to combat chronic illnesses, asthma, diabetes, obesity, and other related illnesses that affect, at a higher degree, more minority populations. We would like to see, I believe, more research done, not in a vacuum, not in just one office, but spread out throughout NIH, so that there are different calibers of individuals and researchers that can provide new, innovative information, so we can combat these illnesses, and hopefully, look at ways of prevention, and making that service available in languages and culturally competent, meaningful ways that will actually make a difference for our populations.

There are no party lines when you talk about healthcare access in communities of color that many of us represent in the House, so I would hope that you would keep an open mind, and work with us, the Members of the Congress, to see that we really achieve parity, in terms of eliminating disparities amongst our communities that currently are faced with some severe challenges and a crisis in healthcare.

So thank you very much.

Mr. DEAL. I thank the gentlelady. Anyone with opening statements? Yes, Ms. Baldwin.

Ms. BALDWIN. Thank you, Mr. Chairman, and thank you, Dr. Zerhouni, for joining us again. I enjoyed our discussion when you appeared before this committee's Health Subcommittee back in March, and look forward to it continuing today.

Biomedical and behavioral research that is conducted at or coordinated by the NIH is of utmost importance to all of America, and particularly, in my district, which includes one of the Nation's leading research institutions. I applaud the chairman's focus on this important part of our government, and I hope that, given the size and the importance of NIH, that we do take a thorough, thoughtful, and measured approach to NIH reauthorization.

Now, I have some concerns surrounding NIH reauthorization, and some of those concerns have been amplified with the circulation of the discussion draft last week. As I expressed at the subcommittee's hearing in March, I have observed ongoing and recently heightened efforts to politicize science and the conduct of research, and I believe that we have to insist upon safeguards to prevent this, and certainly, the time tested peer review process must be protected at all costs.

I just want to end by noting that, while it is a delight to have you return to the committee, I do hope that we will have further hearings on this important topic with some of the other stakeholders that are involved in NIH reauthorization, especially researchers, research institutions, and patient groups.

Thank you, and I yield back, Mr. Chairman.

Mr. DEAL. Thank the gentlelady. Any other opening statements?

[Additional statements submitted for the record follow:]

PREPARED STATEMENT OF HON. PAUL E. GILLMOR, A REPRESENTATIVE IN CONGRESS FROM THE STATE OF OHIO

Thank you Mr. Chairman for holding this hearing and bringing before us a discussion draft aimed at reauthorizing the National Institutes of Health (NIH).

Very briefly, our last NIH revamp bill was enacted 12 years ago, and we must continue to focus carefully on the current organizational, funding, and management structure of the NIH in order to make significant headway in reauthorizing and improving its 27 medical research institutes and centers. We must ensure that the NIH continues to meet our public health needs as well as embrace cutting-edge scientific opportunities.

I welcome Director Zerhouni, and again applaud Chairman Barton's initiative. I yield back the remainder of my time.

———

PREPARED STATEMENT OF HON. JOE BARTON, CHAIRMAN, COMMITTEE ON ENERGY AND COMMERCE

Thank you, Dr. Zerhouni, for testifying once again before the Committee. And I thank all of the organizations and Members who have expeditiously responded with constructive feedback to improve the first discussion draft we distributed last week.

It's time for us to do our job and have the Energy & Commerce Committee reauthorize the National Institutes of Health. This job is critically important and long overdue. With great fanfare, we doubled the budget of NIH. Unfortunately, NIH did not have the mechanisms in place to either account for the increases or strategically apply them. It still doesn't, and that must change.

To date, NIH continues to lack the capability to track dollars across institutes and centers for particular types of research or by disease categories. Only authorizing legislation can put in place the long overdue management tools that NIH needs to provide rational accountability to an agency that needs efficiency as much as it needs money.

I strongly believe that the NIH could be better organized to achieve its mission. This sentiment is shared by many. Nearly two decades ago, the Institute of Medicine reported, when NIH was 10 units smaller and had a budget of $4.5 billion— less than 15 percent of the size of the President's FY06 budget request for NIH— that there should be a presumption against the creation of new research institutes. The alarm bells sounded and Congress ignored them. NIH has grown like topsy-turvy and now there are 27 Institutes and Centers.

Let me be clear. I don't have a problem with the research programs at the institutes and centers. I'm not looking to cut the budget of NIH, nor weaken the fundamental role that the individual institute and center directors play in fulfilling their research agendas. But someone needs to be in charge of strategic planning for the agency. No one in his right mind would ever design a $28.5 billion agency that is fragmented 27 ways with a director with only limited control.

Dr. Zerhouni is certainly to be commended for the job he is doing with the power he can currently exercise. In three years time, he has put in place new management mechanisms to advance cross-cutting, interdisciplinary science. Congress can help Dr. Zerhouni to move forward with these initiatives by moving forward a reauthorization bill.

It's time for this Committee to recognize that it has serious responsibilities with respect to this agency. We can't simply require NIH to conduct more research by spending more money; we must demand that NIH achieves more with taxpayer funds. The status quo is simply unacceptable. On that note, I would like to personally thank Mr. Dingell and Mr. Brown for their help in moving forward this legislation. As I said months ago, the NIH enjoys bipartisan support, and the bill to reauthorize it should be bipartisan as well.

The bill that is the subject of this hearing today was drafted with two key policy principles in mind: no institute or center at NIH would be favored, nor would the bill pick and choose disease winners and losers. I ask my colleagues to keep these important principles in mind as we move forward to improve the bill.

Instead, the bill provides a framework for NIH scientists, not politicians, to identify areas of emerging scientific opportunity and take action to improve public health outcomes. The discussion draft creates a new, comprehensive electronic reporting system that will, for the first time, catalogue all research activities of the NIH in a standardized format. Instead of thousands of pages of reports from each of the research institutes and centers, the NIH Director will compile biennially a report that comprehensively lays out the strategic plans and research activities of the agency.

The bill will let the NIH Director direct by establishing a formal strategic planning process for the entire research portfolio of the agency that transcends the research planning activities of individual Institutes and Centers.

And finally, the legislation streamlines how we fund research activities at the NIH. Science has changed, and so too must the agency that funds it.

By reauthorizing the NIH, we are once again recognizing the critical importance of the biomedical research enterprise that will lead to the next generation of medical breakthroughs and therapies. I look forward to working with Members of this Committee to see that this long overdue bill moves not only through the Committee, but is enacted into law.

Mr. DEAL. If not, we will then proceed with Dr. Zerhouni. We are, once again, pleased to have you here, and look forward to your testimony.

STATEMENT OF ELIAS A. ZERHOUNI, DIRECTOR, NATIONAL INSTITUTES OF HEALTH

Mr. ZERHOUNI. I am very honored to be here, Mr. Chairman, and members of the committee. I think this is probably a defining moment for NIH. There are transitions that are occurring in science as we speak. There are transitions in the way science is conducted, and this topic requires the attention that you have exerted over the past 2 years with 11 hearings. This is my seventh appearance. I have submitted a written statement, and to leave ample time for both comments and questions, what I would like to do is summarize my comments through a slide presentation, if I may.

Clearly, what we are trying to do here, all of us, is to find a better way for NIH, a way that in no way implies that NIH has not been a highly performing organization. In every measure, whether it be GPRA plans or progress in science, or breakthroughs, or impact on public, I think we can say that NIH has been a remarkably successful organization over many, many, many years.

It is important to also remember that our basic authority comes from the PHS Act, Section 301, which states that the Secretary shall conduct in the service and "encourage, cooperate with, and render assistance to other appropriate public authorities, scientific institutions, and scientists in the conduct of, and promote the coordination of, research, investigations, experiments, demonstrations, and studies relating to the causes, diagnosis, treatment, control, and prevention of physical and mental diseases and impairment of man."

And I think what the committee is doing is to reinforce this fundamental authority. We are the primary Federal agency authorized by this committee to conduct and support medical research, and I think the efforts that we are seeing have also been, in many ways, summarized in this list, where, in fact, the basic authorities do allow us to prioritize research at NIH through fundamentally an organizational structure, Institutes, Centers, that are created for special purposes related to perceived scientific opportunities or public health priorities.

It mandates biomedical research, it provides grant-making authority. It mandates a system of peer review which is the envy of the world. It is a world-renowned system that ensures that quality science is funded on a competitive basis. It mandates training for the workforce that we need to address the problems we are dealing with. It also mandates dissemination of information, that the information we generate be made public, and be made available to the public who funds that research, even subject to protections as well, as a wide solicitation of the public advice.

And I think the draft that is being circulated reinforces these authorities, and maintains them, and I want to comment and say that, to me, this is the most important set of reaffirmation of the success of the agency by reaffirming its fundamental authorities. It is clear, however, as the Institute of Medicine study, entitled "Enhancing the Vitality of the National Institutes of Health: Organizational Change to Meet New Challenges," said that "while the NIH is to be celebrated, success alone does not answer fully the question of whether there is a better way to proceed."

Particularly, as one faces a future where the world of biomedical science is being rapidly transformed in virtually all its dimensions. I would like to take a second. There is a quote on the wall there that says: "Where there is no vision, the people perish." Proverbs 29:18. And I think this is what the IOM and your committee, and our own community, have been indicating. If, indeed, there is a transformation, and there are different priorities, how do we set those priorities? What is the organizational challenge we need to tackle as we go into an era of biomedical and behavioral and social science research that is characterized by much more complex problems, problems that affect an entire population at times, problems that affect an aging population, conditions that have become more chronic, more long-term, than the conditions we dealt with 30, 40 years ago. You can survive cancer today. You can live with cancer as a chronic disease. You can live with AIDS as a chronic disease. You can live and survive heart disease for many, many years. The landscape has changed, and I think we need to adapt as well.

Now, at the March 17 hearing, this chart was highlighted by Chairman Barton as illustrating both the opportunity and the challenge that we have. Clearly, as any successful organization, we have grown in size, we have grown in complexity. To the same extent, the complexity and scale and scope of the public health problems we have to deal with have also grown. And as I said, the organization of NIH is primarily an organization driven by structure. So how did we evolve the structure; 27 Institutes and Centers represent the operating arms of NIH, what I refer to as the fingers, if you will. The palm, on the other hand, is represented by some of the coordinated offices, which you see at the top left hand corner, the offices that have been created for the purpose of better coordination, the Office of Research on Women's Health, the Office of AIDS Research, the Office of Behavioral Social Sciences Research. So as you can see, as time has gone by, more structures have been created. But at the same time, we have attempted to create what Representative Ferguson mentioned as the palm. And I think the balance between the palm and the fingers is really our challenge. A strong palm with no good fingers is not a good hand. Strong fingers without a palm is not a good hand either.

So I think going forward and analyzing the proposed circulation draft, these are some of the observations that we can make. I think if you really look not in the structural way at NIH, but in the functional way, what you find is you have Institutes that are specifically directed to research and science that addresses either a disease or a disease process, or an organ, the Heart and Lung Institute, or a particular disease, like diabetes, or a life stage, childhood, or the aging population. These are what I call vertically oriented institutes that integrate all of the components of research needed to address a particular problem, as identified through our public health priority stance.

These are the 15 Institutes that support research specific to either a disease, an organ, or a life stage. Now, any complex organization cannot work when there is only a vertical orientation of each structure. In fact, other Institutes have, for function, research, and science that is just as valuable as the what we call mission specific Institutes, but it supports what applies to all diseases, all organs, all life stages. For example, every discovery at the National Human Genome Research Institute applies to the entire aspect, the entire spectrum of challenges NIH has. We were talking about cross-cutting issues. These Institutes really perform the function of cross-cutting science, and cross-cutting issues like minority health, for example. Basic science, the National Institute of General Medical Sciences, performs science that applies to the entire set of diseases, ages, conditions, organs of the human body.

At the same time, as I mentioned, in the top left corner, there are five program coordination offices that are specific to particular areas of the portfolio. When you think about organizations like this, you also have to realize that as the landscape has changed, what also happened is that with chronic diseases, patients are not affected by one disease at a time, or one organ at a time. They are often affected by multiple failures involving multiple organs. Diabetic patients may have a vascular problem, a neurological problem, as well as a problem of metabolism. So, it is important to realize that barriers and silos become, in themselves, both instruments of effectiveness, but also, instruments by which you lose effectiveness, if you are not able to create that glue.

So I think the concept, the committee's conceptual framework, is a good one. It is truly going from structure, and enhancing that by a functional analysis of what NIH does. However, the one piece that I believe is important is to create the ability for the NIH, on a prospective basis, to analyze its portfolio, to have a real radar as to what is it that is being done within the agency, what is it that needs to be done, that no single institute can do, and what kind of coordination can you accomplish, and how do you accomplish it? And how does it impact budgets? Do you want to direct all research from such an office? No. Centralization is counterproductive in science, excessive centralization, too much top down research. Do you want to have no coordination? Well, the answer is no. Somehow, somewhere, I think the committee is proposing a structure that will accomplish this goal, which is very parallel to what the IOM recommendations have been, and very parallel to what my own actions have been on the ground, when we try to develop trans-NIH programs, such as the Roadmap for Medical Research, or the Blueprint for Neuroscience, or the Trans-NIH Obesity Plan. This OD division would be essentially supporting the glue mechanisms, the coordination—not dictate, but enhance and synergize research. It will include the five specific program coordination offices, which will continue their roles, because they were created to fulfill a gap, which was coordination, and I think they need to continue to do that job.

So in summary, I think you can see that going from a structural organization to a more functional organization does make the case that an authorization structure that would encourage, rather than discourage, integration, that it would encourage synergy, while not losing the autonomy and the ability for the most significant part of the activities of the Institutes and Centers, to be focused on their mission. I think we do see, in my personal view, a great wisdom in what the committee is proposing.

I would like to mention, fundamentally, that NIH and its directors have tried to facilitate cross-cutting collaborations over time. I think it is true that science has changed over the past 12 years, and we have tried to adapt to it. We have adapted to it by an ad hoc process, which I don't think is codified or formalized, and we have shown that it can work, so when we say let us go forward, and make a change, I think I resonate with those who say make sure you don't break the agency. Make sure that what you are proposing works. And I think we have shown that it can work. The Roadmap for Medical Research is one example where all the Institutes have come together, and pooled funds, admittedly, at a time of generous budgets, and have put those funds together to work over a 5-year period, and continue to see this as a valuable initiative. The Strategic Plan for Obesity, or the NIH Neuroscience Blueprint, I think this will accelerate the progress, and make sure that there is, at least, an exploration of a better way.

When you look at the role of this division, I think it will provide consistent analysis across Institutes. It will provide streamlined reporting to Congress. It will provide prospective analysis of emerging areas, either scientific opportunities, like nanotechnology, or proteomics, rising public health challenges, like obesity or any other knowledge gaps can be addressed objectively, on the basis of a transparent and publicly available analysis. I think in conjunction, it should not be done separately from the ICs, in conjunction with the ICs, we should identify the areas that require strategic coordination, where no single Institute can really accomplish the goal that we would like to achieve. And it should launch initiatives that are beyond the purview or resources of any one Institute or Center. High risk, high reward research is difficult to launch when you don't have a common pool of funds that allow you to share the risk. This is, I think, what will serve NIH as a whole.

So we need to make sure that whatever we do does not supplant what has worked, or dictate IC-specific plans. I don't think it is the role of this division to go to the Institute for Cancer and say, "You shall do so." I think it is more important that we stimulate explorations for a part of the portfolio of NIH, to make sure that no stone goes unturned, that if there are opportunities to treat, to make progress, that those are prospectively, in a formalized process, evaluated.

This institutionalized mechanism for allocating a percentage of the total NIH budget for greater synergy is, I think, the core, to me, of the reauthorization concept that I see, which I think would be very valuable. Essentially, it will be a common fund for common needs, with a process that would be, obviously, transparent, that will call for consultation, that will have the right checks and balances for oversight, but at the end of the day, in an era where science has become interdisciplinary, collaborative, and converging in many cases. Most of the research we do at one Institute applies to another. The first treatments for HIV/AIDS actually came from research that was done at the National Cancer Institute. There is no firm separation of good science. There is only good science and good public health.

So in summary, I think that it is clear that the bill, as drafted, does provide, in my view, a higher level of coordination. And I, again, should say that it should not bleed into centralization. I think it should provide input from NIH Institutes and Centers, outside scientists, and the public. It should assess, like I said, a radar of the public health landscape, look at the scientific landscape on a regular and organized and disciplined basis, and manage the NIH portfolio for maximum return on the investment, if you will.

But it will also, in my view, allow something that is always difficult to accomplish in a complex organization, nimbleness, the ability to be dynamic and responsive to quickly emerging opportunities, not wait for the 3 year or 4 year cycle, to be able to address a question, but to be there, on time, with the right amount of money, the right amount of resources, when we need it.

So in summary, I think I am indicating to you a willingness to work with the committee. I think I hear the need for us from the standpoint of policy and national interest, to look carefully at the reauthorization of NIH. We will work with the committee and the staff, in any capacity, to provide the technical assistance that you may wish to have, but, in my view, I think the committee, after 2 years of work, is proposing something that has a functional component to it that does make sense.

[The prepared statement of Elias A. Zerhouni follows:]

PREPARED STATEMENT OF ELIAS A. ZERHOUNI, DIRECTOR, NATIONAL INSTITUTES OF HEALTH, U.S. DEPARTMENT OF HEALTH AND HUMAN SERVICES

Mr. Chairman and Members of the Committee, today is my seventh appearance before the Energy and Commerce Committee or one of its Subcommittees. I have testified about a variety of topics, including research priorities, the organization of Institutes and Centers, scientific peer review, the shift of the Nation's health care burden from acute to chronic diseases, and the need to revolutionize the methods and systems we use to conduct and manage biomedical research.

Each time I testified, I noted the remarkable achievements made in the course of biomedical research, ranging from mapping the human genome to reducing mortality from cancer, AIDS, and heart disease to the rapid progress in the development of vaccines. But I tempered the stories of success by describing the daunting journey that lies ahead of the scientific community as we grapple with the remaining obstacles impeding progress towards the prevention, diagnosis, or treatment of the many causes of human suffering. Much more needs to be learned about human biology and behavior. Emerging and reemerging infectious diseases continue to threaten the world. Chronic diseases are growing in terms of their impact on quality of life and the economic future of America and other countries. The threat of bioterrorism continues to loom. Health disparities remain a widespread problem.

As the Institute of Medicine (IOM) has observed, "While NIH's success is to be celebrated, success alone does not answer fully the question of whether there is a better way to proceed, particularly as one faces a future where the world of biomedical science is being rapidly transformed in virtually all its dimensions."

This quest for the "better way," as the IOM describes it, is also at the core of insuring continued scientific progress in an era when the scale and complexity of the problems we are facing require constant innovation, increased interdisciplinary efforts, and a balanced portfolio of basic, translational, and clinical research investments across all NIH Institutes and Centers. Based on my own interactions with the Members of this Committee, I know you too strive to find the "better way."

The IOM had several key recommendations worth recalling in the context of today's hearing. It recommended that the "Director of NIH should be formally charged by Congress to lead a trans-NIH planning process to identify major crosscutting issues and their associated research and training opportunities and to generate a small number of multi-year, but time limited, research programs." The IOM proposed that NIH present the justification for trans-NIH budgeting to Congress and that the funding for such research should be held in an escrow account. It recommended that such research be included in the President's budget request to Congress for NIH.

The IOM suggested that NIH have a formal process for reorganizing offices and programs.

The IOM also recommended standardizing data and information systems at NIH to enhance management, accountability, and transparency.

The IOM report was followed by three years of analysis by the Committee and its staff. I think it is noteworthy that the IOM and the Committee reached similar conclusions about NIH. Many of these conclusions are manifested in the reauthorization concepts offered by the Chairman and Ranking Member.

In thinking about NIH reauthorization, I want to begin with the core research authorities embodied in Title III of the Public Health Service Act, which authorize the Public Health Service to "encourage, cooperate with, and render assistance to other appropriate public authorities, scientific institutions, and scientists in the conduct of, and promote the coordination of, research, investigations, experiments, demonstrations, and studies relating to the causes, diagnosis, treatment, control, and prevention of physical and mental diseases and impairments..."

I believe this core authority is the fundamental reason why NIH has been so successful in its mission. I applaud the Chairman and Members of the Committee for maintaining these and other vital authorities, such as peer review, the pursuit of scientific opportunity through investigator-initiated grants, human subjects protections, and the requirement to disseminate research findings to the public. In its own search for the better way, I think the Committee is correctly focused on organizational efficiency and effectiveness, which is the principal challenge for an increasingly large and complex organization.

I agree with the Chairman that we should first and foremost carefully reconsider how the organizations of NIH can collectively and effectively support the core missions of the agencies. The challenge is to accomplish this goal through enhanced coordination and partnerships across the NIH Institutes and Centers while avoiding the pitfalls of centralization or top-down research. Achieving the right balance between the necessary autonomy and diversity of approaches represented by the various Institutes and Centers while avoiding the silo effects that can reduce the effectiveness of the whole Agency is the central question. How can the whole be greater than the sum of the parts? As I said in the past, twenty-seven fingers without a palm is not a strong hand. Likewise a strong palm without strong fingers is also ineffective.

I agree with the Chairman that NIH needs an organization, such as the proposed division of program coordination, planning and strategic initiatives, that will serve as a coordinating office for evaluating on a regular basis the progress of science in the context of public health priorities. It will be responsible for analyzing and reporting with consistent methods the portfolios of NIH research that cross the boundaries of multiple Institutes and for identifying trans-NIH research needs that no single Institute can address but that all of NIH needs to support. This structure should be able to conduct appropriate strategic planning for emerging areas of scientific opportunities or challenges and to develop important data and intelligence to support a more comprehensive and informed priority setting process. As you know, the Administration has proposed such an office. I support the concept that this office be able, through a codified process that includes participation from all of the Institutes and the scientific community at large, to allocate resources to initiatives that serve the common good, subject to review by an advisory committee. However, I do not think this office should actually conduct the research resulting from any initiatives it identifies. I believe that this research is more appropriately conducted by the existing Institutes and Centers.

The Chairman also proposes to clearly define the roles of NIH Institutes and Centers. I agree that each Institute and Center should have a defined purpose in support of the overall mission of NIH. The Chairman has proposed categorizing Institutes and Centers into either mission-specific or science-enabling responsibilities. This has resulted in the perception that one category is more significant than another. I understand that this is not the intent. All of the Institutes and Centers support vital research. Some engage in broader areas of science that are useful to all of NIH's organizations while others are involved in more specific areas of research, focusing, for example, on cancer, heart disease, or infectious diseases. Their research is of equal value to the scientific community.

I will work with the Committee to clarify the roles of each of NIH's Institutes and Centers. I agree with his goal of clearly defining how each of these organizations serves the overall mission of NIH and ensuring that the Agency does not consist of 27 silos that do not work in coordination.

In further pursuit of the "better way," the Chairman has proposed consistent coding and reporting of research and a more transparent, efficient mechanism for reporting the results of NIH research to Congress and the general public. I agree that these steps are necessary, and I will work with the Committee to accomplish these goals in a way that will enhance the public's understanding of how NIH works, while not unduly inhibiting the Agency's ability to conduct and translate research quickly.

In conclusion, I pledge my cooperation to work with the Committee as it considers reauthorizing the NIH provisions of the public health Act. I look forward to answering any questions that you might have.

Mr. DEAL. Thank you. I will begin with the questions.

As you know, we are considering in this proposal to divide the various Institutes and Centers into two big categories, one that is mission specific Institutes, and two, the science enabling Institutes and Centers. What do you think about this approach to that two major divisions?

Mr. ZERHOUNI. I think functionally, you can see that the mission is actually different for the two groups. It is really important to have the ability to coordinate planning between these. As I said, for example, you may have conditions and diseases that affect multiple organs. Diabetes affects the cardiovascular system, affects the brain. So you want more coordination around diseases, for example, that go across multiple Institutes that are focused on diseases.

At the same time, in the cross cutting Institutes, that are just as important, you may see an emerging discipline. You may see something that—a methodology, or you may actually want to, for example, develop computational biologists. Well, that cannot be done by any one of them in isolation. So there is, I think, merit to—from the planning standpoint, to have these Institutes make sure that they get coordinated in a way that is strategically directed.

Mr. DEAL. I am sure most of us have heard from groups that feel like they are not adequately represented within the silos that currently exist, and one of the complaints is that they get shuffled from one to the other, that this is not that institute's responsibility, it is somebody else's.

One of the ways that we have anticipated trying to deal with that is through the reporting system that is in the draft legislation. Do you believe that this reporting system is a good way to let the public know what is or is not being done and by whom, and is this an important ingredient in setting priorities for you within the NIH itself?

Mr. ZERHOUNI. First of all, I would like to commend the committee, for looking at this issue of reporting. It is a consuming activity that consumes a lot of resources and staff time, for a benefit that is not necessarily there. So I think streamlining reporting would be of great value to us, and strategically reporting, in an appropriate way, would be important. But think about it. If you had a division like this, that had consistent ways of recording data and information, that across all activities, the NIH had a way, a consistent way, of reporting it dynamically, if you had an issue, you wouldn't have to create a report, or a need for a report. What you would do, you would say this division should be charged to look at, for example, in the case of autism, we developed an autism plan, called an autism matrix, and the case of Parkinson's disease. And the question should be what is in the portfolio, and what is science telling us, or public health telling us, that we are not doing. That sort of dynamic reporting is, I think, the future, but you can't do it unless you have the tool to do it. And I think, with the tools, we could streamline it.

However, I think mandated reports of a very large size, basically, in my view, would be counterproductive. We need to be more nimble. We need to be more accessible. I think someone said accessible public information. That, I think, will solve the problem eventually. So I am in favor of streamlining reporting.

Mr. DEAL. Thank you. Mr. Brown.

Mr. BROWN. Thank you, Mr. Chairman. Dr. Zerhouni, I just have a series of short questions, and I hope that, if possible, you can give pretty quick answers to them.

One of the questions before the committee is whether we include specific authorization levels in a bill reauthorizing NIH. Do you support the committee legislating a hard ceiling, or—a hard ceiling on NIH funding?

Mr. ZERHOUNI. Well, you are creating a real conflict in my mind here. As the Director of an Agency, there is no ceiling that is good enough, but I do understand the necessity for the authorizing committees to look at that issue, and clearly, I think it—like we said, it really depends on the total structure of the authorization bill, and the specific amounts, and so on, over what time. I think the details need to be worked out, and would be happy to talk about the consequences. It needs to be done carefully, if it is to be done.

Mr. BROWN. Well, if we have ceilings or caps, let me push it a little further. If we have ceilings or caps, what is an appropriate percentage increase? What is an appropriate number, if there are those caps or ceilings?

Mr. ZERHOUNI. I think you need to really look at the planning process, and you need to look at the opportunity well. I mean, you can't tell what emergencies will occur, what opportunity will come. So it is very, very important to leave yourself a significant amount of flexibility.

Mr. BROWN. I am not going to get a specific—answers that I want here, am I?

Mr. ZERHOUNI. I am willing to work with the staff and the committee. I think it is something that needs to be looked at in greater detail.

Mr. BROWN. The draft contains several different authorities for the Director to transfer funds within the National Institutes of Health. One of these follows the Institute of Medicine's recommendation that each Institute and Center set aside a percentage of its budget into an escrow type account to be applied toward trans-NIH initiatives, as we discussed, a sort of common fund. What is an appropriate percentage that we should set aside, if we do it in the authorizing language for trans-NIH authority?

Mr. ZERHOUNI. Well, clearly, I think, it wouldn't be meaningful if it is not a meaningful percentage. I think—and I think the IOM recommended beginning with 5 percent of the overall NIH budget, and I think that this is a good way of making sure that the NIH Institutes come together on a regular basis, because this is not transferred away from the Institutes. I think it should stay within the Institutes, but allocated dynamically over a period of time, and the initiatives to which it is allocated should not be permanent initiatives. They should be time limited. If you do that, I think, obviously, you need to have a significant portion, 5 percent is, in my view, a good recommendation as a minimum.

Mr. BROWN. As a minimum.

Mr. ZERHOUNI. For a common fund.

Mr. BROWN. Yes.

Mr. ZERHOUNI. Now, there is a difference between——

Mr. BROWN. You are saying a minimum——

Mr. ZERHOUNI. [continuing] a minimum——

Mr. BROWN. [continuing] or the optimal number, 5 percent.

Mr. ZERHOUNI. I am reading you the——

Mr. BROWN. What do you think?

Mr. ZERHOUNI. I think 5 percent should be a minimum.

Mr. BROWN. Okay, a minimum. Okay. And you want to set it up so that it is not an entitlement, so that it doesn't ultimately lead to another Institute, in effect.

Mr. ZERHOUNI. That is right. I think the idea of creating another structure that has funds, and allocates that to—over an infinite period of time is not the concept. The concept here is to create an organization that will identify what areas to incubate better, what emerging areas need to be supported, what emerging areas need to be funded. But it shouldn't be forever. It should be time limited, and we can discuss how to do that, technically, but I don't believe that those initiatives should live there forever.

Mr. BROWN. And what other kind of transfer authority that the Director, that allows the Director to transfer funds from one Institute or Center to another Institute or Center. My understanding of current law is that you have the authority to transfer 1 percent of any of the Institutes' or Centers' budget in this way. In that 1 percent, that—my understanding, that is what the appropriators have done, have allowed. I am not sure that we have addressed that. Have you made use of that 1 percent transfer as Director?

Mr. ZERHOUNI. Okay, historically, if you look at the use of the transfer authority, because it is an authority that comes post facto, it is not planned ahead of time, and if you know the reality of the budget process, you have to plan at least 2 years ahead of time. We are currently dealing with the 2007 budget, while the 12006 is not done. So what you really need, transfer authority is only used in cases where your planning missed something. Something happened where you need to quickly react to a—something on the ground that is happening in real time, so you transfer small amounts. So historically, the transfer authority has never been used for a prospective, strategic purpose. It is usually reactive and post facto. So the transfer authority doesn't have to be a large authority. The common fund concept, however, needs to be real and significant.

Mr. BROWN. Last question, real quick, Mr. Chairman. On the transfer authority, not the common fund, but the transfer from one Institute to the other. Is the—should the 1 percent number be in the authorizing language? Should it be 2, should it be a half? I understand that you haven't used it—you have used it very infrequently, if at all. What should we do there? Give us a specific number.

Mr. ZERHOUNI. There is no doubt in my mind that it should be in the authorizing language, because not being in the authorizing language makes it unsure.

Mr. BROWN. What should be in the authorizing language, 1 percent, 2 percent, .5 percent, what?

Mr. ZERHOUNI. Again, I will have to think through what the topics are, but 1 to 3 is usually what people recommend, the AAMC says up to 3, the IOM says up to 3. One to me—it depends on what else you have. If you have a common fund that is in law, in authorization, where everybody knows that they have to come to the table, and plan jointly, then the transfer authority can be smaller. If you don't, then you have to rely on the transfer authority, like we did for the Roadmap, for example. The first year of the Roadmap, I used the transfer authority.

Mr. DEAL. Mr. Bilirakis.

Mr. BILIRAKIS. Thank you, Mr. Chairman. Doctor, you have spoken, and I would say pretty fondly, of the committee draft. Obviously, in your remarks, you didn't go into the dollars of it. Mr. Brown did, and I would sort of like to maybe hitchhike on his questioning.

In my opening statement, I was concerned that we not cause any harm, basically, the old doctor's education adage, "Do no harm." In that connection, thinking in terms of multi-year commitments in research portfolios, thinking in terms of longer range planning, which is, I guess, basically the same thing. Thinking in terms of— or politics. Politics sometimes in NIH would be maybe even heavier than politics in Capitol Hill. Ultimately, it is the real world is, I guess, is what I am talking about, the ability to shift funds. Talk about that, in general.

Do you feel that the areas that you have not mentioned, such as the four specific authorizations or appropriations, the competition which is envisioned there, the transfer authority, the increased transfer authority that would be given to your office. I think, even though the legislation is blank, it leaves it open in terms of what that percentage would be. It certainly envisions considerably higher than what your office now holds.

So in terms, again, of the things that concern the—tell us a little—take the rest of my time, and tell us a little about that.

Mr. ZERHOUNI. I think it is a very good area to focus on. From my standpoint, what is really important here is to establish the proper checks and balances, just like our system of government works on checks and balances. There is always the possibility of misdirecting decisions at the executive level, if you don't have the proper checks and balances. And I think the same is true, that you could also have such an entanglement, and such a limitation on what the executive can do that you are not getting an efficient organization. So the answer to that, I think, is what I believe in very strongly. No. 1, complete preservation of the peer review process. No. 2, relying on the input from the Institutes and Centers who are closest to the action, understand the research, and have a process that is formalized, where in fact, that consultation occurs. And third, an outside oversight mechanism such as the Advisory Council of the Director, which is, in law, the mechanism by which all Institutes, really, are overseen, with public members and scientific members.

I don't think it is as big a problem as I think some people are afraid of, but I think it will depend on the details of how you establish the proper checks and balances, so that there isn't excessive authority being exercised on a discretionary basis without reporting back to Congress, and to the appropriate members.

Mr. BILIRAKIS. Well, but excessive authority, sir, and checks and balances and whatnot, I mean, that is pretty darn subjective. It is in the eyes of the beholder, I guess.

Mr. ZERHOUNI. Right.

Mr. BILIRAKIS. And so here, we put ourselves in the shoes of these research facilities out there, and from the standpoint, again, of the multiyear planning, and whatnot. There still would be, in the hands of—basically, right now, of course, they are in the hands of the Appropriations Committee's up here.

Mr. ZERHOUNI. Right.

Mr. BILIRAKIS. They would be in the hands of the Director to a very large degree.

Mr. ZERHOUNI. I think they would be balanced, because no project that the Director can come up with will not—will be accepted without peer review. So all of those will go through that two level of peer review process. Second, if you predicate the ability of having an allocation done for a particular purpose, on the need for a consultation with the Institutes, so that the scan that I am talking about is done, and remember that we are only talking about trans-NIH areas of concerns, where the palm has to be stronger than it is today. I think it is doable. I don't think—it is an achievable goal. Complex organizations do that all of the time. As long as you have a proper oversight structure and the corporate board structures to have enough input.

Mr. BILIRAKIS. You know, over the years, when I chaired the subcommittee, I guess the most terrible times that I had was when I had people coming in to me in wheelchairs or whatnot, and they wanted increases in research funding for that particular, specific disease, and having to tell them that we have a policy here of not basically telling NIH how they should spend that money. So I guess you are making this—if this were to go forward, it probably makes it easier on us, in the sense we would pass the buck on to, I guess, to you, if you—is that correct?

Mr. ZERHOUNI. Well, I hope it is not the intent here, because I would definitely see that as not a good evolution. I think, in fact, the reason our American science is as good as it is, and NIH science is as good as it is, is because of the wisdom of Congress in avoiding specific earmarks independent of the peer review process, independent of that check and balance system that is really the envy of the world. So I would prefer to preserve that, rather than have more coordination, to be honest with you.

Mr. BILIRAKIS. Well, thank you, sir. Thank you, Mr. Chairman.

Mr. DEAL. Thank you. I know that you cannot see the timer. The only thing you can see is probably when the red light goes off at Dr. Zerhouni's table there. And we have a timer up here. The Science Committee is just not as advanced as we are in our committee, but if you would try to watch that timer there, so we can get everybody with questions. Mr. Waxman.

Mr. WAXMAN. Thank you, Mr. Chairman, Dr. Zerhouni, I want to ask you about advisory committees at NIH. The National Research Council of the National Academy of Sciences recently recommended that appointments be made on the basis of scientific and technical knowledge and credentials, and professional and personal integrity. Do you agree with that statement?

Mr. ZERHOUNI. Yes.

Mr. WAXMAN. The National Research Council also stated that it is inappropriate to ask potential candidates for advisory committees about non-relevant information, such as voting record, political party affiliation, or position on particular policies. Do you agree with that view as well?

Mr. ZERHOUNI. Yes, I agree.

Mr. WAXMAN. In recent years, there have been serious allegations made that advisory committee appointments were dictated by politics, and not science. In one well publicized case, an advisor to a panel on drug abuse was asked whether he had voted for President Bush, and whether he supported abortion rights. In another case involving the Fogarty Center on International Health, numerous proposed experts were rejected by the Department for apparently political reasons, and those rejected included a Nobel Prize winner. Would you support clear language adopting the National Research Council's standards as guiding advisory committee appointments at NIH, and essentially saying the NIH Director would make appointments without political interference by the Department, these appointments should be based on scientific merit, not political litmus tests, and Congress should remove any temptation to meddle with this process?

Mr. ZERHOUNI. Well, when I became Director I looked into them. The NIDA case, for example, that was not a department selection with NIH. You are talking about a Nobel Prize Committee member. I understand that same person is now an advisor to the Office of Science and Technology Policy. I have heard a report from one member, who had been asked questions like this. So——

Mr. WAXMAN. Whatever happened in the past—in the future, do you think it would be a good idea to write that into the language?

Mr. ZERHOUNI. Let me just say this, Congressman, that to my knowledge, since I was aware of that one case, and I intervened no one on any NIH council, peer review or advisory, is unqualified to be on that council. So I want to make sure you know, my commitment is to, in fact, achieve that. And during my tenure, there has not been——

Mr. WAXMAN. Dr. Zerhouni, I am not really being critical of you. I am just asking for questions on this legislation. Do you think we ought to write that in?

Mr. ZERHOUNI. By and large I think NIH is—should be apolitical. I think it is apolitical, I think disease knows no politics. I think we should really advise and inform, and do the research that serves the entire country, and do it in the most objective way possible.

Mr. WAXMAN. You have been a strong advocate for NIH's system of peer review of grants, and its independence from political pressures. Do you believe the NIH Director should be able to defund a grant that has passed peer review by an Institute?

Mr. ZERHOUNI. I think there would have to be really, a very, very scientifically justified reason to defund it. We do have cases where there are issues of integrity of the science, misconduct, where we have to defund. So the NIH Director needs the authority to defund, but not on the basis of a political decision.

Mr. WAXMAN. Well, the reason I ask is that the idea has been floated to make the NIH Director responsible for eliminating unnecessary, duplicative research, and for ensuring balance in research. I understand the need to constantly——

Mr. ZERHOUNI. Well——

Mr. WAXMAN. [continuing] review NIH's research portfolio, to make sure it is responding to the challenges facing the American people, but I am concerned about giving any Director, a political appointee, you know, broad authority to second guess the scientific experts to rate the grants in their fields. What should be the NIH Director's role in assessing the portfolio——

Mr. ZERHOUNI. I think priorities, in my view, should be allocated and priorities means resource allocation, at the end. I think——

Mr. WAXMAN. But not micromanaging.

Mr. ZERHOUNI. Not micromanagement. You should really do it on a prospective basis. For example, we allocated resources, greater resources, to the obesity issue, that you know well, prospectively. Once it goes to that level, I think the Director should trust the peer review process, and not second guess a two level process. The peer review process, two levels of independent review is the cornerstone of NIH, and why it has been successful. So prospectively, doing priority setting, absolutely. Changing the relative weights, because science changes, and public health priorities, absolutely. Retrospectively, I don't think it is a good idea.

Mr. WAXMAN. Thank you. Thank you, Mr. Chairman.

Mr. DEAL. Chairman Barton, do you have questions?

Chairman BARTON. Mr. Chairman, I am going to defer at this point in time, to kind of get a feel for the hearing, but—the Energy Conference is in recess for 30 minutes, so before I go back downstairs, I would like to be called on. But I want to study up a little bit right now.

I am glad to know where all my energy conferees are, though. They are all up here at the NIH hearing. But I am going to defer at this point in time.

Mr. DEAL. All right. Ms. Wilson.

Ms. WILSON. Thank you, Mr. Chairman, and thank you, Doctor, for being here to testify.

I had a couple of questions. I had a particular interest in this issue of managing research portfolios, which I think is very different than a lot of the other things that we manage in government. And I am interested not in what are the best opportunities for research and science, but how do you determine what are the best opportunities? What tools do you have as a Director, or within and across your Institutes, for determining what the best opportunities are?

Mr. ZERHOUNI. Of how it is done. So fundamentally, about 60, 65 percent of the budget is allocated to what we call scientifically-initiated proposals, so it is investigator-initiated proposals, a scientist out there has a great idea. They submit the idea to the peer review process, which is the first step at the top, is the NIH grant proposal. It then goes to a scientific review panel. And only 25 percent of these get ranked to be funded, and it goes through the program officer. Now, the program officer in each Institute follows a particular strategic plan, that has been usually developed over a period of years by the Institute, to look at program importance and program relevance. And that officer will determine whether or not the grant fits with the program relevance of that Institute. And then, it goes to the second level of review, which is the Institute National Advisory Council, and that Institute has, in law, in statute, the authority to fund this research or not fund it, and sometimes, they will change the priorities at that level. And this goes to the Institute Director, reported back to Congress, obviously. This is the issue of reporting that we cover.

So this is done at the level of the Institutes, and the ability of the NIH in total to combine all these portfolios is limited. This is why, I think, this reauthorization strategy will provide the ability to look across Institutes and across portfolios. And Institutes have done that on their own, and many Institutes have come together to look at areas that are common. Usually, with a lead Institute serving as the disease-specific need. So the process seems complex, but there is no doubt that within each Institute, planning is done, has always been done, in a very effective way, and the Program Directors, in conjunction with the Advisory Councils, will then determine what the portfolio will be for that Institute.

What you don't have, as effectively as we—what I believe we should have, is a look across all portfolios, with analytical tools that tell you how much are you spending in this area of research versus that one. And duplication is not necessarily bad in research. You need to confirm findings. You want to have that. But it is the balance, is the issue of what is the right balance.

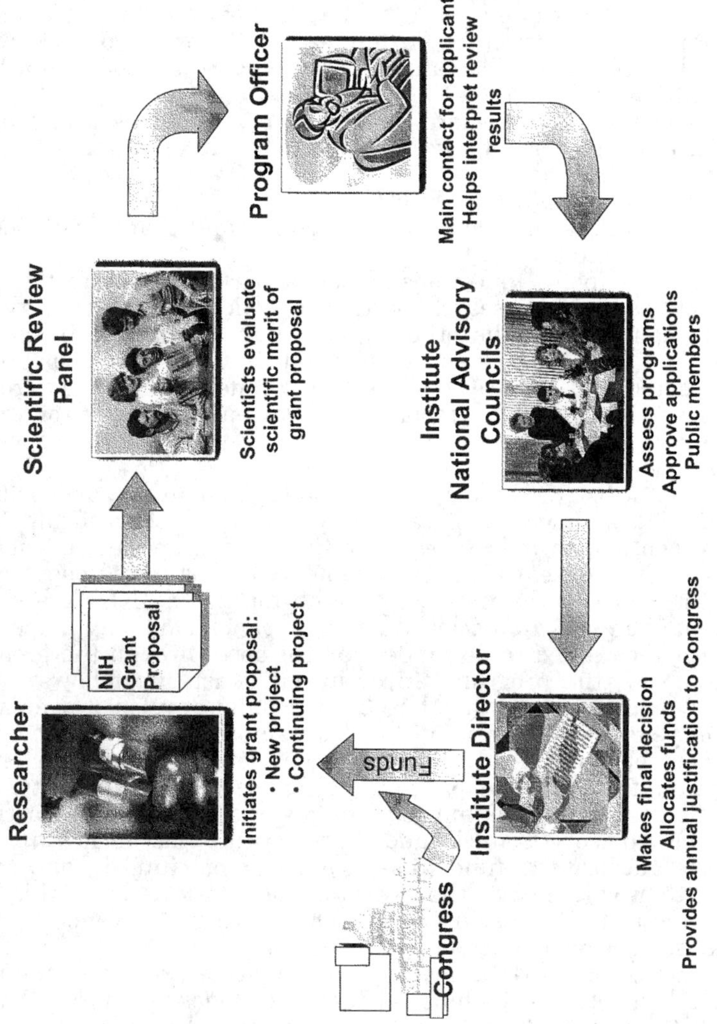

Ms. WILSON. I find that interesting, that it seems to be driven from the bottom up, from the researchers. There may be some value to that. At the same time, you as a Director need to be——

Mr. ZERHOUNI. Right.

Ms. WILSON. [continuing] looking at what are the biggest problems.

Mr. ZERHOUNI. Right.

Ms. WILSON. [continuing] that we need to identify research roadmaps, and gaps in research in order to fill. And that is—is there anything that you currently have that does that kind of an assessment of here are the biggest health problems, whether it is the cure for diabetes, which is driving health costs, or aging problems? Do you have any mechanisms to do that?

Mr. ZERHOUNI. Actually, my answer was incomplete. Sixty-five percent of the budget is allocated to investigator initiated proposals, and about 30 percent is allocated to what we call requests for applications, or requests for proposals, or contracts, where we identify, ourselves, an area where further investments are needed, or an action is needed, or new Centers are created. We put those announcements for competition to the field, and that is how we balance the portfolio between what comes from the bottom up, and what we want to get accomplished. I am sorry, I missed that.

Ms. WILSON. I will be interested in pursuing that, as we move along here on reauthorization. And finally, I just ask for your thoughts on how to structure a system to give access to research, and whether you think it should be public, or only to medical practitioners. Should it include the successes as well as the failures? What are your thoughts on how you would pursue this?

Mr. ZERHOUNI. This is a topic that we discussed entirely with NIH Directors as well as scientists, and it is a very major component of the Roadmap for Medical Research, where in fact, we think that we should make investments in information technology that would be accessible at the community level. We think that we need to train community practitioners in research methods, and have a core of 50,000 community practitioners that would have access to our data base, called clinicaltrials.gov, where we are listing about 14,000 clinical trials. I think we need to enhance the ability for us to link those trials to the results of those trials.

So my view is more openness, more transparency, more access, to community physicians in particular, because chronic diseases are seen in the community much more so than they are in academic health centers. And we have an initiative, which will start this year, called Clinical and Translational Science Awards, which we are going to announce at the end of August, September.

Mr. DEAL. Ms. Eshoo, you are recognized for questions.

Ms. ESHOO. Thank you, Mr. Chairman, for holding this very important hearing, and welcome, Dr. Zerhouni.

This is a very large undertaking. I have been in the Congress, this is my thirteenth year, and I am always thrilled when we get to reauthorize NIH, which I always like to refer to as the National Institutes of Hope, and I think that is the way the American people view the NIH, and it is in that spirit that I ask the following questions.

First, on transfer authority. This transfer authority is thought to allow you, the Director, and succeeding Directors, more flexibility to run projects and to streamline the budget decisions, but of course, we don't want flexibility to undermine any accountability. And I raise this because last year, broad transfer authority was given to the NASA Administrator, and I think with devastating consequences. I have a major NASA Ames, maybe it is good that we are the science hearing room—someone may come off the walls on this. I have a NASA facility in my district, NASA Ames, right in the heart of Silicon Valley, and we saw that budgets were being realigned not to spur progress and development, but to cover funding shortfalls in other areas.

So it was—that transfer authority was being completely, I think, misused, and I know that there isn't anyone here that wants to see transfer authority misused. What would you suggest that could be built into the reauthorization, with these proposed changes, that would not allow the NASA, you know, the—what I just described happening at NASA, to happen within the NIH?

I want to ask my questions, then you can answer. I mean, I agree that NIH scientists are, by and large, more equipped than Congress on where—maybe so, you know, as a partner, on how best to spend the money, where it should be directed. But I am concerned that scientists would not have any kind of role in the transfer authority. I think when the—let me just summarize it by making this observation. I think NIH works best when it is collaborative. I don't think it was ever meant to be an institution that has such a powerful Director that there is only one conductor of the orchestra. You have to have someone that leads, but I do think that the collaboration needs to be built, and so that it is enjoyed across the board. As you explained, I mean, we have entered a new era. So this transfer authority business is a bit troubling to me, if it is not handled right.

And I have concerns that dividing the NIH Institutes and the Centers into two categories will not necessarily make NIH function more effectively, or improve Congressional oversight of appropriations. And on that key word of, in terms of appropriations, I know it is a tough call for you to make, but you know what the needs of the agency are. I am highly skeptical of doing reforms anywhere, when they are meant, they are really—it is really dressing the issue up to cut or to not fund properly. And you know, one doesn't take the place of the other. In fact, reforms, many reforms can't be carried out unless you have the necessary resources. I see where the FDA is having a very tough time. FDA has not been funded properly by the Congress, and yet, we have so much that we expect from the agency. So if we are going to live up to National Institutes of Hope, and the changes that are afoot, what would you instruct us about transfer authority, so that it is what it should be, and not what I described happening in another agency.

And also, on the organization of Institutes, you know, there was one that I helped to found. I don't know if it is—with this plan, it is going to be wiped. I mean, I have had people come to me and say it is working very, very well, the Biomedical Imaging and Bioengineering Institute. So if you would comment on my observations also my questions, I would like to see a good, healthy appropriation for NIH. It is only to help to make the changes, but we have to—this century is going to be the—is going to be known, I believe, as the century of the biomedical changes. And if NIH is not embraced by the Congress, in terms of an appropriate appropriation, then it is going to be—we are going to be talking about out of both corners of our mouth.

So take it away.

Mr. ZERHOUNI. Well, very important points. I think the——

Mr. DEAL. You have 30 seconds to respond.

Mr. ZERHOUNI. Okay. That is——

Ms. WILSON. He can respond—for the committee as well.

Mr. ZERHOUNI. Yes, I can certainly respond, but I don't think——

Ms. WILSON. They are serious questions.

Mr. DEAL. Just looking for the question mark.

Mr. ZERHOUNI. As a Director I think it is important to remember what I said before, and that is, it is the balance that is key. A dictatorial counselor authority wouldn't work, and I would like to just read, I think, one of the recommendations of the IOM report, which captures what I think is trying to be accomplished here.

"The Director of NIH should be formally charged by Congress to lead a trans-NIH planning process"—everybody is at the table—"to identify major cross cutting issues in their associated research." That is collaboration, because think, not having any such authority removes the accountability of the Director to be able to direct the agency to what it needs to do. So there is a balance between the two. The question is where you find that balance. And it does instruct the Director to present the scientific rationale for trans-NIH budgeting to the relevant committees of Congress, including a proposed target for investments in trans-NIH initiatives. So it is not a transfer. It is a common fund for common good, for common needs. That is the concept. And I don't think it should be deviated from that, provided we put the right checks and balances and transparency in it. That, I believe, is needed by the NIH.

Mr. DEAL. Dr. Burgess.

Mr. BURGESS. Thanks, Mr. Chairman. I will be glad to yield to the full committee chairman, if he——

Chairman BARTON. If the gentleman doesn't mind, I appreciate that.

First, Dr. Zerhouni, thank you for testifying today, and thank you for you and your staff's efforts working with us the last year, as we have worked with the stakeholders to come up with the legislation, the draft legislation, that we are looking at today. I want to let the committee know that this is a very high priority for me as chairman. If we wish to reestablish the authorizing committees in a meaningful way, when overseeing the agencies that we theoretically have jurisdiction. Under the current environment, we haven't reauthorized NIH in 12 years, and in all—to be totally true about it, most of the oversight that is being done is being done by the appropriators. So this effort, while you can argue with the specifics of the draft, is an attempt to reassert the jurisdiction of the authorizing committees in general, and the Energy and Commerce Committee specifically over one of the more, if not the most, one of the more important agencies in the Federal Government.

We have—as well as we all know, we have doubled the budget of NIH, but we have not done anything to try to help their management structure, or help them come up with a mechanism for allocating all these new grants and funds that we have provided them. Nothing in the current draft legislation in any way denigrates the peer review process, the two step solicitation, the grant process at NIH. Nothing. We keep our hands off of that. We are not trying to micromanage. What the draft does do is collapse the 26 line items to four, No. 1, give the Director, in this case, Dr. Zerhouni, more direct authority, by empowering him, and enlarging the—his direct discretion, and then two, creating this trans-NIH fund, that is multi-agency with NIH, and give it real budgetary authority, and real dollars, so that as we have these cutting edge ideas come forward, they are looked at across the NIH, concurrently, as opposed to individually within each of the 27 Institutes.

I think that is a very good idea. So my first question to you, Dr. Zerhouni, the general concept of going from multiple line items, in this case 26, down to a more, a smaller number, in this case, four, at least in approach, do you support that? If you don't maybe support the exact numbers, do you support the principle?

Mr. ZERHOUNI. Again, I think, as I testified while you were busy with the other committee, Mr. Chairman, I believe that the approach, the conceptual approach you have taken in bringing functional integration, through the mechanism of identifying what is the function, relative to the structure is, in my view a good approach. The details, obviously, of how you implement that on the ground, and how do you play that, it is obviously something we need to work on. But I think the fundamental concept, that the agencies become more complex and larger, and needs to be more efficiently managed through a transparent process that makes people have a common good, a common fund for a common good, overall, this is, in my view, a good contribution to the agency.

Chairman BARTON. What about the line item that we would create, that is trans-agency, that we give direct authority, with a discrete amount of money, that it would allocate funds across the different Institutes.

Mr. ZERHOUNI. My comments to that are, Mr. Chairman. I think you need what I call an opportunity fund. When something comes up that is actually critical, you need the ability to house it somewhere, so that you can implement it quickly at the time of the budget request, and that it be authorized. So that is what I call the opportunity fund.

Then, I would say that it is important to have a trans-NIH fund of some sort, called, what I call the common fund, where everybody is incentivized to come around the table and discuss, without being afraid of, essentially removing from their own specific mission resources, because they are mandated by the authorization language to say you need—you shall come together, and you shall identify what is cross cutting, and what needs to happen. So the authority for having an opportunity fund is important, because you never know what comes up. For example, biodefense came up, and we need to react to that.

A trans-NIH fund is certainly a necessity, and some transfer authority. It doesn't—if you have those two, you don't need large transfer authorities, because they are different in nature. Transfer authority is post facto. A trans-NIH fund is prospective. So I think the combination of these three is really what would make the agency work well.

Chairman BARTON. My—I see my clock has expired. I want to ask one more question. As we put the draft out for review, there appears to be a lot of concern about where we would set the baseline, the first—if we—if this bill were to become law, where we would set the baseline. Now, my preference would be that the first year, if this bill were to become law as-is, the baseline for each Institute would be whatever the funds that it received in the prior year. So we would guarantee every Institute, you know, that—100 percent as the baseline, and then, we would start from there, and you could go up, and—or they could go down, but the very first year, every Institute would be held whole, and then we would begin this internal review and internal competition, and with your discretionary fund, and the trans-NIH fund, in terms of the first year's baseline, is that your view, too, that each Institute would start at 100 percent of last year's funding?

Mr. ZERHOUNI. Well, clearly, as you know, the process of science is not something you can do over 3 months, stop, and start again. So it would be very important to make sure that you don't disequilibrate the system, I mean, the agency does work relatively well. To the extent that you—and I would certainly echo what you just said. I mean, it would be very important to preserve the, you know, the momentum that many of these Institutes and Centers have undertaken. What I think is important, also, is to realize that the—depending on how we—you technically settle on what is common fund, what is opportunity fund, what is—then, the answer will affect, obviously, what you wish to accomplish through that mechanism of putting, I think, a floor.

I think it depends on that planning process.

Chairman BARTON. Okay. And I want to thank you, Dr. Zerhouni. I also want to thank the chairman of the Science Committee, Mr. Boehlert, for allowing us to use his hearing room, the Science Committee hearing room, so that we could continue our markup at the Energy Conference downstairs. And if we have energy conferees here, not to name names, but Mr. Stupak and Mr. Bilirakis, to name a few, we are—and Mr. Wynn, we are reconvening in 10 minutes downstairs.

Thank you, Mr. Chairman.

Mr. DEAL. Mr. Wynn came in late. We are still confused as to why he is sitting over here, Mr. Chairman.

Ms. DeGette, I believe you are next.

Ms. DEGETTE. Thank you very much, Mr. Chairman.

Dr. Zerhouni, we have been told by the leadership of this committee that what they are really trying to do with this NIH reauthorization bill is to look at the organizational structure, and see if there are ways—in a bipartisan manner, that we can reauthorize the bill by looking at the structure, and looking at some of what I think are your very wise suggestions. I agree with that approach for the most part. I think—I mean, I have many fabulous pieces of legislation which are bipartisan, that I would like to see included in this bill, but I am going to try to work with the leadership. But there are some questions I have been sitting here mulling over, listening to the testimony, and listening to the questions of my colleagues on the panel, and I am wondering if you can comment a couple of these. It is not about do we need more research for this or that, or—tempting as—though it may be, stem cell research.

Instead, I was thinking about when you talked early in your testimony, and it is this slide here, which your staff kindly provided me with, the key authorities that the NIH has, prioritizing research, mandating biomedical research, providing grant-making authority, mandating peer review, mandating training, mandating dissemination of information, mandating human subject protections, and mandating the solicitation of public advice. Do you think all of those areas should be included in a reauthorization of the NIH?

Mr. ZERHOUNI. Yes. I think those are the basic authorities, and they have served NIH very well.

Ms. DEGETTE. And I would agree with that. But really, in your view, when we do this reauthorization in the committee, we should try to work in a bipartisan way to look and see if the NIH current mandate is adequate in all of these areas, and whether it can be beefed up or expanded or improved, correct?

Mr. ZERHOUNI. The privilege of the committee, absolutely.

Ms. DEGETTE. Okay. The reason I ask that is, I have a particular interest, which you know. In this list of items, in the human subject protections, and as you know, Dr. Zerhouni, I have been working previously for many years with Jim Greenwood, who was the previous chairman of the Health Subcommittee, and also, I have talked with Mr. Barton and other members about human subject protections. I am wondering if, in the draft legislation, you or your staff expanded the human subject protection authority that the NIH currently have, as—or have you addressed this at all in the draft? I haven't had time to really delve into it.

Mr. ZERHOUNI. Not to my knowledge, but I certainly will check. I have not personally focused on that issue, but certainly, we would be more than happy to share with the committee staff what the status of human subject protection is, and—in the context of what I know you are interested in.

[The following was received for the record:]

The NIH has a long-standing commitment to the protection of human subjects of research that dates to the first formal policies it developed for its intramural program when the Clinical Center opened in 1953. Since then, through Congressional directive and Executive initiative, the agency has developed a comprehensive network of standards and requirements so that NIH-sponsored research, both intramural and extramural, meets the highest levels of human subjects protections.

The legal authority for NIH oversight of human subjects protections in research supported or conducted by the NIH derives from the Public Health Service Act, which at 42 USC 289 directs the Secretary of Health and Human Services to establish oversight of research conducted or supported by HHS and its agencies. In accordance with this legal authority, research supported or conducted by NIH is subject to federal human subject protection regulations, known as the Common Rule, found at 45 CFR part 46, subpart A. These regulations require informed consent and IRB review. HHS regulations that specifically concern protections and considerations for pregnant women, fetuses and in vitro fertilization, as well as prisoners and children can be found at 45 CFR part 46, subparts B, C, and D. These regulations are referred to as the "Common Rule" because the federal government, in June 1991, published them as a common policy for federal agencies conducting or supporting research with human subjects. Today, it governs seventeen agencies and most federally-supported research. Additionally, when NIH-funded research is regulated by the Food and Drug Administration (FDA), it is subject to FDA's human subjects regulations incorporated at 21 CFR parts 50 and 56.

NIH has measures in place to help ensure that NIH-funded clinical research complies with the ethical guidelines and regulatory requirements for research involving human subjects and that the rights and welfare of human subjects participating in NIH funded studies are protected.

For the NIH intramural program, a distinct office is charged with helping intramural investigators understand and comply with ethical and regulatory requirements for research involving human subjects. In the extramural program, NIH has regulations and policies in place to help NIH-funded clinical research comply with the ethical guidelines and regulatory requirements, including 45 CFR part 46, for research involving human subjects.

Pursuant to its authority to set the terms and conditions for research that it funds, and consistent with the requirements of 45 CFR part 46, the NIH has implemented specific requirements for the protection of human subjects in research that it funds or conducts (see generally 42 CFR part 52). These include:

- A requirement that applicants or offerors describe and justify the risks to the subjects, the adequacy of protection against these risks, the potential benefits of the research to the subjects and others, and the importance of the knowledge gained or to be gained;
- The evaluation of proposed human subjects protections by peer reviewers and NIH staff, and appropriate resolution of human subjects issues before the study can be initiated;
- Confirmation that the institution has a current Office for Human Research Protections (OHRP) "Assurance" on file attesting to its compliance with 45 CFR part 46;
- Certification of review and approval of the research by an Institutional Review Board (IRB) registered with OHRP under the institution's Assurance.
- Education in the protections of human subjects for research study personnel designated as "Key" to human subjects research so that they understand the underlying philosophy and specific requirements of human subjects protections when engaged in clinical research; and
- A plan for data and safety monitoring for all NIH-funded clinical trials; the NIH policies specify that the level of monitoring should be commensurate with the risks and the size and complexity of the clinical trial. For certain types of studies (phase III and many multi-center trials), the monitoring must involve a group of independent experts called a data and safety monitoring board (DSMB). The role of the DSMB is to review accumulating safety and outcome data in order to help ensure the continuing safety of current trial participants and those yet to be recruited.

These requirements are included in the NIH Grants Policy Statement, which is a standard term of award for grants and cooperative agreements. These requirements are also incorporated into research contracts. An NIH Institute or Center also has the authority to include additional conditions on the award for specific studies (see 45 CFR part 52.9). Also, because of special risks and societal concerns, trials involving human gene transfer that are conducted at or sponsored by institutions receiving NIH funding for recombinant DNA research must be registered with the NIH. Investigators responsible for those trials must report adverse events and other pertinent information to the NIH, as outlined in Appendix M of the *NIH Guidelines for Research Involving Recombinant DNA Molecules.*

Ms. DeGette. Yes, because a couple of things I am interested in with the legislation, I am interested in, for example, the common rule, which now applies in all research that is funded by the NIH, but does not necessarily apply in other types of research. Am I correct?

Mr. Zerhouni. I am not totally briefed on this, and——

Ms. DeGette. Okay.

Mr. Zerhouni. [continuing] current, but I think you are right.

Ms. DeGette. And I am wondering if this might be an area that we could explore in a bipartisan way, beefing up the application of the common rule more broadly, into research that is either directly or indirectly affected by the NIH activities.

Mr. ZERHOUNI. Be happy to, you know, to work with the committee——

Ms. DeGETTE. Okay.

Mr. ZERHOUNI. [continuing] and the staff, your staff, to look at that. Obviously, the Office of Human Research Protection at the Department also has jurisdiction over that.

Ms. DeGETTE. Exactly. Right.

Mr. ZERHOUNI. So you have to look at that issue.

Ms. DeGETTE. Okay. But that is certainly a topic that you think would be appropriate in the NIH reauthorization bill. Thanks, Doctor, and I yield back.

Mr. DEAL. Thank the gentlelady. Dr. Burgess.

Mr. BURGESS. Thank you, Mr. Chairman.

Dr. Zerhouni, when you were here earlier this year, I think one of the things that came up was the—when we restructured the intelligence agencies last year, one of the big discussions around town was if you don't have the budgetary authority, then you don't have the authority.

Do you feel that this reauthorization that we are doing currently, does it provide you with the budgetary authority that you need in order to exercise the appropriate authority over the NIH?

Mr. ZERHOUNI. I think the important component of the reauthorization is this ability for the Director to have an instrument by which all of NIH comes together, for at least a small portion of the total budget, and looks at what I call the glue areas, the synergy areas. That is an important institutionalized process that needs to happen for any complex agency. That would provide that.

In terms of budget area, currently, obviously, the Director can always make an administration budget, and through interaction with the department and OMB, present a budget to Congress. That authority is there. But typically, what happens is everything goes in lockstep, and the reason it goes in lockstep is because of all of the stakeholders and different pressures and programs that you have, unless there is an emergency, or something that changes the equilibrium. What I am talking about is instead of having this, is to look at a small layer of the budget, and plan it together, not dictate or direct it. I don't think the NIH is an agency—it is a knowledge organization. You really need to manage it according to that.

So I think the reauthorization will provide marginal budget authority for a very specific purpose, but overall, the budget authority in the current authorization does allow you to make some marginal changes, but not a lot.

Mr. BURGESS. I must admit, when I first looked at that organizational chart that you showed us early in the year, and knew that we were coming to this reauthorization, my feeling was that there would be significant consolidation between the various departments, and I guess I won't say that I am disappointed that there is not some consolidation, because after having been onsite, and watched some of the great work that you do, I realize how little Congress should, in fact, meddle in the system that you have. But do you feel that there is enough along the lines of consolidation in the organizational chart that you maintain with this reauthorization?

Mr. ZERHOUNI. I think this allows for a greater degree of functional consolidation that is not there today. I don't think it allows for structural consolidation. I think structural consolidation does happen over time, as science will—changes. I think a reauthorization, in my view, should be done regularly. It shouldn't be a one time event every 12 to 15 years. So I think we should really look at this, and see how it works, and adjust in 3 years time. I don't think this is an impractical proposal, but I do believe you need to show that you have the mechanisms of functional integration, before you can go ahead and destroy structure, and combine structures in a way that may not be productive.

Mr. BURGESS. The—Ms. Wilson, who was here a minute ago, talked about the ability to get information to the public, and I must admit, after 20 odd years in clinical practice, I did not know about clinicaltrials.gov. Maybe there is an opportunity there to do some public service announcements to medical societies across the country. I thought I saw the AMA here earlier today. That would be, I think, a good thing, because I can remember times, being in the treatment room and being absolutely baffled about what do I do next. It would have been great to know that I could have gone online and gone to clinicaltrials.gov, and gotten that rare cucumber virus tended to.

And then, finally, I just can't help myself. What do you see on the horizon, looking over the horizon, as some of the new scientific areas of study that your organization may be working on in the near future?

Mr. ZERHOUNI. Dr. Burgess, you should see the progress we are making. Every month, there is a new discovery, a new breakthrough. Recently the National Cancer Institute reported on a research study that showed that by looking at 16 cancer-related genes, in women who have breast cancer sensitive to estrogen hormones—you know, in the past, we had about 100,000 women with that, and all of them underwent surgery and chemotherapy. By looking at that—those 16 cancer-related genes, you can see that 70,000 of these women will not benefit from chemotherapy, whereas the other 30,000 do. So that research is going to completely transform the way we practice medicine in the next year or 2, and we will save about $8,000 per year of treatment, because we will avoid chemo, unnecessary chemotherapy. And I think that is the trend. We—a month before that, we reported in Science and PNAS, three of our grantees discovered a gene for age related macular degeneration, which will affect 7 to 10 million Americans over time, that will lose vision because of this. We never knew what the cause was until this research, but it has to do with a blood protein called Factor H, and no one had any clue that this could have come from not your eye but your blood. So this is a breakthrough that is going to make it possible for us to prevent blindness in the aged population. The acceleration and the momentum that I think we have been able to demonstrate with the funding that you have provided us is, in my career, remarkable, my own personal experience. I have never seen such a rapid fire of discoveries that can really change the way we practice medicine.

Mr. BURGESS. I appreciate that. Could you give the committee just a little flavor of what is the magnitude of scientific throughput that is required to come up with one of these genetic determinations?

Mr. ZERHOUNI. I see—I can see you really enjoyed the briefing, sir. Basically, that is the key. The key, for example, the cancer research, they looked at 250 genes in thousands of patients, put that into a large data base, analyzed the data base through a high throughput system, come down on to 16, then did trials on thousands of women. So it really is a scale and complexity that required more than the NCI itself could do, but multiple collaboration. So that is the trend, interdisciplinary, collaborative, large scale, but yet, still, coming from the scientists, and bottom up, rather than control and—command and control.

Mr. DEAL. Ms. Baldwin, would you defer to Mr. Stupak. He is just dying to get back to the conference committee, I can tell. I will come back to you, if you will do so. Mr. Stupak.

Mr. STUPAK. Thank you, and thank you, Ms. Baldwin, for yielding.

Dr. Zerhouni, you mentioned that the need to ensure clinicaltrials.gov is accessible as possible, and that results of trials are also accessible as possible. Do you support the making the results mandatory, having them published?

Mr. ZERHOUNI. Basically, we do believe that it is important to connect clinicaltrials.gov to what we have been trying to do through public access publishing, so that any report that comes out in the public domain be linked, so that when someone looks at clinicaltrials.gov, they know what that trial, what the results of that trial eventually were. So I think we are in favor of more transparency and more reporting, and more registration of all trials. The issue of whether or not you can do reporting on the fly about adverse events or other things, that needs to be looked into, because it goes beyond our jurisdiction. That is an FDA issue, but yes, we are in favor of trials being connected to their results in some fashion, and accessible to the public.

Mr. STUPAK. Do you have subpoena power to information that you might find interesting in these trials?

Mr. ZERHOUNI. No, I do not.

Mr. STUPAK. You talked a lot about the fingers and the palm of a hand, and how do you get the information you need from these trials that raise a flag with you, if you don't have any——

Mr. ZERHOUNI. If it is a trial that is——

Mr. STUPAK. Yes, I am sorry. Enforcement power.

Mr. ZERHOUNI. If it is a trial that is funded by NIH, we have, obviously, the mechanisms to look to what we call a data monitoring and safety board, which is an independent board that looks at what the investigators and what we are funding. That is how, for example, we reported on the issue of Celebrex in a trial of the National Cancer Institute, and other trials that we were looking at. So for NIH funded trials, we have authority——

Mr. STUPAK. Well, how about non-NIH funded?

Mr. ZERHOUNI. With non-NIH funded trials, we have no authority. We are not a regulatory agency. The FDA does.

Mr. STUPAK. So you may be aware of clinical trials that may be detrimental to human health, but if they are not published, you really can't have access to them, to check the credibility, or their—any evidence.

Mr. ZERHOUNI. We have access to our own, and when—and as I said publicly, our threshold for stopping a trial is, obviously, greater than—I mean more sensitive than others, because we are doing research, so we never know that there is a defined benefit. The FDA is the agency charged for regulatory oversight of other trials.

Mr. STUPAK. Right. Well, as I said in my opening, both you and the FDA have this responsibility to make sure we have sound clinical trials to protect the health and safety of the American people, but neither one of you have any kind of subpoena power, so how do you enforce it? What——

Mr. ZERHOUNI. NIH——

Mr. STUPAK. Well, take Celebrex. You mentioned it yourself. There were other trials out there you knew of, but you didn't have access to them, because they weren't your own. So how do you obtain that information?

Mr. ZERHOUNI. NIH does not have subpoena power, but I am not an expert on the regulatory——

Mr. STUPAK. FDA doesn't either—that is fine.

Mr. ZERHOUNI. I think that is—I haven't thought about that question, of how you connect the enforcement powers with the oversight powers. I would be happy to come back on record for you.

[The following was received for the record:]

NIH has access to safety information for the clinical trials we fund. In addition, NIH policy requires data monitoring in all clinical trials and, for certain types of studies, depending on stage, level of risk, design, and organization, the monitoring must involve a group of independent experts, called a data and safety monitoring board (DSMB, see *NIH Guide for Grants and Contracts,* June 10, 1998 and June 5, 2000). The DSMB's role is to review accumulating safety and outcome data in order to help ensure the continuing safety of current trial participants and those yet to be recruited as well as the continuing validity of the trial.

Safety information on clinical trials funded by the private sector must be reported to the FDA when those trials are conducted as part of the development of drugs, devices, or biologics and data is intended to be submitted to FDA for regulatory approval purposes (see 21 CFR parts 312 and 812). NIH does not have direct access to adverse event information about such private sector trials. However, we work closely with FDA and are able to factor information FDA makes publicly available into our own decision-making about the continuing safety of clinical trials we support and conduct. In this regard, our work will be aided by FDA's efforts to ensure that established and emerging drug safety data are quickly available in an easily accessible form. In addition, we have established a working group to help consider and, if necessary, make improvements in our assessment and response to emerging safety information from clinical trials or in post-marketing product surveillance that has implications for NIH clinical studies and study participants. The goal of the effort is to ensure that NIH's response to such events is timely, coordinated and well considered.

We are also working on longer term efforts to promote greater transparency and awareness through enhanced clinical trial registration and access to published articles and results summaries in ClinicalTrials.gov, NIH's database of clinical trials. In establishing ClinicalTrials.gov, Congress mandated the registration of all treatment trials subject to FDA regulation, regardless of funding, that address life-threatening and serious diseases and conditions (see 42 USC 282(j)).

Mr. STUPAK. Sure. It has always amazed me that the—some of the regulatory agents, like FDA and—not that you are necessarily a regulatory agency, but when you are responsible for basic health needs, you have no power to get the information you need to help make the decisions.

Mr. ZERHOUNI. Except for what we fund.

Mr. STUPAK. Except for what we—you fund, right. And while we wish you had more money, it is not all the money that is going into research. There is a lot of research out there.

I mentioned in my opening the importance of one program, pediatric research, and the consequences of striking its authorization. Is there anything else in the committee draft that may have been stricken that you would like to see? What is missing in this committee draft that you would like to see, besides subpoena power?

Mr. ZERHOUNI. Any special authorities that were removed, you mean?

Mr. STUPAK. Yes.

Mr. ZERHOUNI. Well, that is—I haven't really thought about what was removed that would be of critical importance. I think—I am not sure what it is that I would—I am just thinking through as—think, but——

Mr. STUPAK. Sure. Sure.

Mr. ZERHOUNI. Can I get back to you, and look at that, specifically?

Mr. STUPAK. One more, since my time is just about up. How are we doing on the flu vaccine for next year?

Mr. ZERHOUNI. We, just last week, had the results of the first phase of our clinical trials. As you know, NIH has gone forward in developing a vaccine on H5N1, which is the variant of the virus that we suspect will be the—if it mutates to the point of becoming transmissible. We have good results. There is a dose response we know we have a vaccine. Now, we need to go to the other phase, but we are very, very pleased with the Phase I results.

Mr. STUPAK. Thank you, and thank you, Mr. Chairman, for your courtesy.

Mr. DEAL. Thank you. Mr. Ferguson.

Mr. FERGUSON. Thank you, Mr. Chairman. Dr. Zerhouni, I apologize. I have been out, as I know a number of other members have been. So I may have missed if you have addressed some of these questions.

Mr. DEAL. Well, we have all been here. We have all been here.

Mr. FERGUSON. Yes. You, Mr. Chairman, I know, have been here. We talked—I talked a little bit about, and you have referred to the 27 fingers—you need the palm. In your review of the draft, do you feel like we have—the draft adequately addresses your need, as the Director, or the need of any Director to properly coordinate what is going on, to provide the adequate palm, if you will, for management purposes?

Mr. ZERHOUNI. I think it is a good draft, and I think we need to clarify some details. As I said, I don't know if you were here, I said 27 fingers without a palm is not a good hand, but a strong palm with no fingers is not a good hand, either.

Mr. FERGUSON. Right. Right.

Mr. ZERHOUNI. So we need to find the balance between the two, but I think we are getting there, and I think the committee staff and the committee draft are going in the right direction.

Mr. FERGUSON. And if you have, obviously, as you are talking about, some of this, specifics or the details, I am certain that we will be talking with you further as you have advice or thoughts, input for us as we continue to go through the process. I hope you will.

Mr. ZERHOUNI. I will certainly do that.

Mr. FERGUSON. Wouldn't you share that with us? Like Mr. Stupak, I am particularly interested in childhood diseases, as well, and I think it is—I feel strongly that we need to make sure that our agencies are really working together properly, and working toward research on diseases for, frankly, one of our, probably our quietest constituency is our kids. How do you feel like this draft, and as we are—the direction that NIH may be heading, and how will that improve your ability, with regard to the cutting edge research, and translating that research into actual cures, for some of the childhood diseases that we have talked about?

Mr. ZERHOUNI. As you know, the fundamental authority of NIH allows NIH to do research in every field, including pediatric research. I believe that having an instrument like this division of program coordination is going to allow all of us to prospectively, rather than retrospectively or after a lot of lobbying, to understand what disease process is doing what, to truly prospectively look at the evolution of childhood diseases of particular concern. I think that, to me, will be the result of a modern reauthorization bill that would institutionalize not only the mechanism but the obligation to look at the landscape of public health for children, or for any other population.

Mr. FERGUSON. And will further enable the agencies to, and the Institutes to kind of get out of their silo, to get out of their, perhaps, more narrow, necessarily narrow view?

Mr. ZERHOUNI. Well, I think the Institutes have done a good job when it came from their specific mission needs. I think we should really not think that the Institutes have not collaborated. The Roadmap is a collaboration. What I think I am talking about is when there is an area of science or public health where no Institute has either the resources or the expertise, or the ability, if you will, to look across, and this is where, I think, that would be very helpful.

Mr. FERGUSON. Well, I—these are just a couple of the points that have been kicking around in my head.

Mr. ZERHOUNI. Right.

Mr. FERGUSON. And I think a number of the points that some of the others on the committee have raised today are equally important. So I appreciate very much your insights and your advice, and not only your work at NIH, but as we go through this process, looking to the future, your continued input is going to be very important for us, so we appreciate very much your time today, and——

Mr. ZERHOUNI. Thank you.

Mr. FERGUSON. Chairman, I yield back.

Mr. DEAL. Thank the gentleman. Ms. Baldwin.

Ms. BALDWIN. Thank you, Mr. Chairman.

I have, first, a narrow question, and then some broader questions on reauthorization. In your testimony, you talked about the mission specific division relating to research around disease or organs or life stages, versus what has been called the science enabling division, having more cross cutting issues. And I just looked at the list of Institutes that would be congregated, as proposed in the draft, I noticed that the National Institute of Environmental Health Sciences, is under the disease, organ, and life stage specific grouping. I wonder if you could tell me a little bit more about what is happening in that Institute, so I could derive whether that is an appropriate placement of that institute, versus the other divisions that it could be possibly placed under?

Mr. ZERHOUNI. I have to say that you are very observant, and I—we have been——

Ms. BALDWIN. Well, thank you.

Mr. ZERHOUNI. [continuing] actually, thinking about the NIEHS being, again, as—if you look at the fundamental definition, does research in NIEHS apply to all organs, all disease, all life stages, and the answer is yes, so you could think of NIEHS being a cross cutting Institute.

Ms. BALDWIN. We will take—I am sure we will take a closer look at that, and have greater discussion.

On some broader questions, with the establishment of four specific appropriation line items for NIH, that we have gone over what those are, I am concerned about the impact that lumping the Institutes and Centers, most of them in two line items, will have, in terms of pitting them against each other for the available funding. In a worst case scenario, you would see a competition that would result in the loss of cross-institutional collaboration and cooperation that we have recently enjoyed. I wonder if you could comment on that, and talk about ways to prevent the pitting of institutions against each other, what we might want to have as safeguards in this legislation to prevent that.

Mr. ZERHOUNI. That is a very good question. The way you structure a reauthorization structure drives culture. Structure drives culture, and therefore, you can't really look at that issue in isolation. You really look at the total structure that I think is being envisioned here. There is no doubt that losing the identity of a mission is not necessarily a good thing, so you need to find balance between the two, and clearly, you don't want to have a zero sum game that occurs. You really want to, therefore, have what I call a common fund for common good, for funding when there is a need to do it. But again, I mean you have programs that sometimes don't need to move out of a particular Institute to be coordinated with another Institute. So to me, the most important thing is to keep the planning process, the ability to present a logical plan to Congress, to the—I mean to Congress in general, and the appropriators in particular, that keeps that identity for the mission. Otherwise, what you end up with is no one is responsible for anything. So you need to strike that balance between the two.

Ms. BALDWIN. Are you comfortable with legislation that places a limit on the number of Institutes in each division? Right now, I think they are looking at 15 in the mission-driven, and nine——

Mr. ZERHOUNI. There is no doubt that, you know, the way Institutes and Offices and Centers have been created has been, I wouldn't say haphazard, but frankly, driven by factors other than pure science. I do believe that, you know, there is a particular law in—that every time you add one, you double the complexity, and every time you add another one. I think it is not a good idea to have so many structures, and I do believe we need to have a limit, and if anything, think about reorganizing. I was just reading the New York Times this weekend, and General Electric went from 11 divisions to six. And obviously, it is a completely different environment, completely different, but we do need to have a limit to the number of direct reports and units that are independent, that duplicate their own administrative structures and so on. So yes, I think every observer, including the IOM, by the way, would say you need to be very careful in adding any. I think we should subject all of this to a public process, as recommended by the IOM, but I do believe that limits are a good thing. If—we need to have the discipline of recognizing a mission, but not at the expense of complexity of management, and unwieldiness of the agency.

Ms. BALDWIN. Dr. Zerhouni, I see that amber light, which means my time is almost done, in fact, I think it is done, but there are two questions that I want to pose, and you don't have to answer right now. They are both following on questions previously asked by Mr. Waxman and Mr. Brown.

First, there is the blank by the authorized appropriation level. Any guidance you can provide us, in terms of how we should be considering opportunities as we deliberate over what the optimum rate of increase for NIH is appropriated, and second, following up on Mr. Waxman's questions, whether we should have specific language in this draft, or in the final bill, for the next Director of NIH, who will be a political appointee, to direct them in terms of composing the advisory committees and the institutes?

Mr. ZERHOUNI. I will submit my answer in the record.

Ms. BALDWIN. Thank you.

Mr. DEAL. Thank the gentlelady. Mr. Buyer.

Mr. BUYER. I want to cover a couple of questions. One, in particular, that deals with your Roadmap, and a followup off of Mr. Ferguson's question that he had to you about how this legislation, will it really permit you to implement your Roadmap? And so that I can understand that better, I think anyone that wants to take on an organization like—that you have—functional consolidations of an organization, to integrate activities, to meet strategic goals based on priorities, that is noble. I—that is your job. That is what you want to be able to do. And as I was listening to you testify, I was thinking about a couple years ago, you came up, and you testified about your Roadmap. A lot of us got pretty excited. I remember asking you a question about sexually transmitted diseases in America, and I was pretty stunned—correct me if I am wrong, but I thought your testimony was that there are 80 million Americans, is that about right? Or 65 million?

Mr. ZERHOUNI. Sixty-five million, growing by 4 million a year.

Mr. BUYER. Wow. Sixty-five million Americans have been infected with a sexually transmitted disease. If you actually—take of our population of 295 million people, and say of that population, then, what is the highest in sexual activity, you are almost looking at a one in three, one in four perhaps.

Mr. ZERHOUNI. This is—lifetime, yes.

Mr. BUYER. Yes, in a lifetime, have dealt with a sexually transmitted disease. And the reason I remember that is because you, then, said Congressman, this is an epidemic. All right. It is an epidemic. I would think that is an epidemic. If you think about it, our society, and this is a problem that—it is sort of the problem in the closet. It is sort of the problem in the basement, a problem that nobody really wants to talk about somehow, until we have to deal with it. So I look at this, and you could pick a disease. It doesn't have to be a sexually transmitted disease, but I brought that up, because I remembered you talking about it, and I look at you now trying to do this consolidation. You have got your Roadmap, and—so my specific question for you would be can you give us some actual examples from your experience on how the current individual Institute and Center-oriented structure of NIH, or limited authorities results in missed opportunities, or significantly impeded your ability to respond to opportunities and public health challenges, such as the one that you called the epidemic?

Mr. ZERHOUNI. Right. That is a very good question. You have seen the example of the Roadmap. The Roadmap was not designed to address any particular public health challenge—it was really the first time that all Directors said, "We really need to do better in cross-investment." So they came together, and if you look at, I think I have this—this is the investment of the Roadmap.

[The following was received for the record:]

Roadmap Funding

dollars in millions

	FY04	FY05	FY06	FY07	FY08	FY09	Total
Pathways to Discovery	64	137	169	182	209	188	948
Research Teams	27	39	44	92	96	93	390
Clinical Research	38	61	120	174	214	227	833
Total	130	237	332	448	520	507	2,172

Directors Fund   35   60   ??

-All NIH ICs and NIH director have made the corporate decision to create a common pool of resources that will be used for all current and future investment in the Roadmap initiative

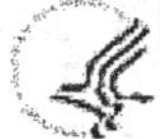

Mr. ZERHOUNI. We decided to have three topics, pathways to discovery, research teams, clinical research, things that we identify as gaps in our investment, and commit to a 5-year process. Now, at the time, funding was a lot easier. It is about 1 percent of the NIH budget, over time. But when you were done with this, what you realize is that you hadn't been necessarily responsive to obesity, for example. So the next year, we asked Dr. Allen Spiegel, from the National Institute of Diabetes and Digestive and Kidney Diseases, Dr. Nabel from the National Heart, Lung and Blood Institute—at the time, Dr. Lenfant, to come up with a trans-NIH plan on obesity. That is how it works, but you know what? We never really had the mechanisms or the idea of having a process that would be prospectively looking at that. And I have been trying to instill this in my interactions with the agency, because I do believe, from my previous experience in the private sector, that science requires that now. It is too complex, but you need to have a crosscut of exactly what you are doing.

So what other opportunities? Neuroscience. If you look at the disease burden in patients from 25 to 44, mental health becomes the major problem that affects the population, drug and addiction, alcohol abuse, behavioral problems, neurodegeneration, and mental health. You take those five, it is a $500 billion healthcare cost. So we decided to have a Neuroscience Blueprint this year, which we are presenting in 2006, but guess what? You couldn't fund it, because there was no prospective mechanism by which you would say here is a set aside fund. This is our opportunity fund. This is our common fund. Let us just make sure that every time there is an emergency out there, that we react to it. So the question you are asking is, this will provide you a mechanism to look at public health burden, what is rising, what is not rising. We knew about obesity all these years, but we really didn't have a mechanism to A, plan for it, and then, allocate resources. The mechanism that usually happens is an office is created in law, like the Office of AIDS research, because there is a public health emergency, or this is more language that is put in the bills, because a particular disease process or constituency wants that served. I think having this process would continuously allow NIH to be responsive, nimble, and proactive.

Mr. DEAL. Thank the gentleman. Mr. Rush.

Mr. RUSH. Thank you, Mr. Chairman.

Dr. Zerhouni, the last time that you appeared before our committee, the question that I asked was what could NIH do to better promote the inclusion of minorities and women in clinical research, both as subject and researchers. And can you tell us now how exactly NIH dollars are being used to promote racial and gender inclusion, and also, include in your answer whether or not NIH dollars are being used to promote minorities and women as researchers themselves, and also, included in your answer, would you give us some idea about how can NIH encourage private sector companies, such as pharmaceutical firms and medical device manufacturers to include minorities and women in their clinical research, as both subjects and also, as researchers? Can you give me a quick answer on those, please?

Mr. ZERHOUNI. Well, first of all, let me say that if you have attended some of my presentations, health disparities is one of our top five priorities, and remains one of our top five priorities. No. 2, there are two parts to your question. One is what are we doing in terms of having a scientific workforce, a medical workforce, that is able to study and research these conditions? Our basic philosophy is that, from the scientific standpoint, it is very clear that the diversity of those who conduct the research has to mirror the diversity of those who participate in the research as subjects. So we have this philosophy that to penetrate communities, you have to be there, and you have an interaction that is constructive with a diversity that reflects that population. That is a challenge, because when you look at the number of women or minorities in science careers, what you find is difficulties there. I mean, it is an opportunity issue. Young African-Americans, for example, who are very successful, may not necessarily see science as a maximizing opportunity for their own career. On the other hand, I think NIH has been consistently proactive in building minority training programs. The new Center on Minority Health and Health Disparities spends quite a bit of resources on building the infrastructure for that, and you can see it is paying off.

The other issue is participation. That is an issue that relates to the Roadmap, and the concept that you need to conduct research at the community level. So we funded, for example, the Jackson Heart Study. The National Center for Primary Care that Morehouse has funded, with 136 community centers, having a presence in the communities. That is the answer. The answer is you have to be on that ground, with trained people that are connected to all the trials that are ongoing, if you really want to have participation.

Mr. RUSH. I want to quickly move to another one of my interests. A Newsweek magazine that highlights the problem of uncertainty within the medical profession when it comes to prescribing drugs for children. According to the article, because drug companies have not invested in clinical research involving children, apparently, it is not very profitable, the doctors are basically flying blind with nothing but speculation when prescribing drugs to children. The results can lead to both inadequate treatment and even death, and Mr. Chairman, there is an article that I would like to submit for the record, a Newsweek article that I would like to submit for the record.

Dr. Zerhouni, what should NIH do to correct this problem, and what can Congress do to ensure NIH is addressing the problem, and is the solution including children in clinical trials?

Mr. ZERHOUNI. Well, as you know, the BPCA, the Better Pharmaceuticals for Children Act, mandates that we look and rank all of the medications that need testing in children, because we do believe that we need, there is a need for making sure that we understand how—what is the dose, what are the side effects, which may be different. So we have a process through the National Institute of Child Health and Human Development, that looks at the drugs. There is a committee that meets at the departmental level, and in conjunction with the Foundation for NIH and the FDA, essentially prioritizes the trials that need to be undertaken in particular—

adult drugs that are used for children. So we have a mechanism, and I think that mechanism leads to——

Mr. RUSH. Well, how effective is that mechanism? Because we still have a very serious issue, and a serious problem with children who are getting inadequate dosage, or maybe too much dosage?

Mr. ZERHOUNI. I know it is, can I get back to you on that, because I know we have about 11 drugs that are being tested, or on the list of being tested, but I don't know the specifics at this point.

[The following was received for the record:]

DEPARTMENT OF HEALTH AND HUMAN SERVICES

National Institutes of Health

National Institute of Child Health and Human Development

**Report on Progress In Implementing The Best Pharmaceuticals
For Children Act**

Elias A. Zerhouni
Director, NIH

March 2005

DEPARTMENT OF HEALTH AND HUMAN SERVICES

National Institutes of Health

National Institute of Child Health and Human Development

**Progress In Implementing The Best Pharmaceuticals
For Children Act**

Table of Contents

Executive Summary 1
Introduction 2
Background 3
Funding for the BPCA 3
Studies Initiated During FY 2004 3
Drug Development Process 4
Collaborative Efforts Utilized to Initiate Drug Studies 4
On-Patent Drugs 5
The List Development Process – FY 2004 5
Preparing the Priority List for January 2005 6
Need to Expand Knowledge Base 7
Conclusion 8
Table 1: Projects Funded to Date with Yearly and Estimated Total Costs 8
Table 2: Drug Studies Initiated During FY 2004 9
Table 3: Drug Studies Proposed for FY 2005 10
Table 4: Drugs Reviewed at the 2004 Scientific Meeting and Recommended for Inclusion
on the 2005 List 10
Table 5: Status of Remaining Drugs for the 2005 Priority Listing 11

**Progress In Implementing The Best Pharmaceuticals
For Children Act**

Executive Summary

In their reports on the FY 2005 budget for the Department of Health and Human Services, the Senate and House Committees on Appropriations recognized the importance of ensuring that drugs are safe, effective and appropriately labeled for pediatric use. Both Committees requested an update describing the number of studies; estimated cost of each study; the nature and type of studies undertaken; the number of label changes resulting from completed studies; the patent status of the drugs studied; and the number of drugs remaining on the priority list. The following is submitted in response to these requests.

In 2004 NICHD began the third cycle of the development of the annual list of off-patent drugs prioritized for study in children. Our experience has demonstrated that much more information is needed about medications used with children, and the conditions for which the medications are used. To ensure the widest public health benefit, the NICHD is more fully emphasizing data regarding frequency of use by children and the indications for such use in identifying drugs for study. Additionally, NICHD has developed initiatives to access and synthesize data on medications used by outpatient populations as well as data regarding inpatient medication use.

In FY 2004, six off-patent drug studies were initiated. In FY 2005, an additional five studies are planned, including studies of four off-patent drugs and one on-patent drug.

Industry experience indicates that it will take approximately five years to complete a pediatric study and submit data to FDA for a labeling change. To date, no clinical studies have been completed to allow for a labeling change. When the clinical study is completed, the data will be submitted to the FDA for review with the intent of modifying the label to improve pediatric therapeutics.

**Progress In Implementing The Best Pharmaceuticals
For Children Act**

Introduction

In its report on the FY 2005 budget for the Department of Health and Human Services (DHHS), the Senate Committee on Appropriations stated:

> "The Committee recognizes the importance of ensuring that drugs are safe and effective for use by children and are appropriately labeled for pediatric use. The Committee strongly supports continued implementation of the Research Fund within the National Institutes of Health, as established in the Best Pharmaceuticals for Children Act of 2003 (Public Law 107-109) within section 409I of the Public Health Service Act, which supports the pediatric testing of off-patent drugs, as well as on-patent drugs not being studied through existing mechanisms. The Committee urges NICHD to act as the coordinating Institute for other Institutes within NIH for which pediatric pharmacological drug research may have therapeutic relevance, and urges consultation with the Food and Drug Administration to ensure that the studies conducted through the Fund are designed to yield improved pediatric labeling. The Committee expects an update prior to the fiscal year 2006 hearings, including information on the number of studies supported through the Research Fund; the estimated cost of each study undertaken; the nature and type of studies undertaken; the number of label changes resulting from completed studies; the patent status of the drugs studied; and the number of drugs remaining on the priority list established through section 409I". (Senate Report No. 108-345, page 129)

Similarly, the House Committee on Appropriations in its report on the FY 2005 budget for the DHHS stated:

> "The Committee recognizes the importance of ensuring that drugs are safe and effective for use by children. The Committee supports continued implementation by NIH of the Best Pharmaceuticals for Children Act of 2002 to support the pediatric testing of off-patent drugs, as well as on-patent drugs not being studied through existing mechanisms. In implementing this responsibility, NICHD should act as coordinator for all other institutes within NIH for which pediatric pharmacological drug research may have therapeutic relevance. NICHD is also encouraged to consult with the Food and Drug Administration to ensure that the studies conducted are designed to yield improved pediatric labeling. The Committee requests NIH to provide an update during its annual appropriations testimony on the number of studies supported; the estimated cost of each study undertaken; the number of label changes resulting from completed studies; the patent status of the drugs studied; and the number of drugs remaining on the priority list. NICHD should focus its resources on encouraging the study of drugs where there is a medical necessity to conduct clinical pediatric studies, consistent with ethical concerns. The Committee also urges NICHD to give full consideration to existing information that supports the safe use of drugs in children and use of conditions contained in the Pediatric Research Equity Act to identify drugs for study and to determine the scope and magnitude of those studies". (House Report No. 108-636, page 108)

In response to these requests, the National Institute of Child Health and Human Development (NICHD) of the National Institutes of Health (NIH) prepared the following report.

Background

The Best Pharmaceuticals for Children Act (BPCA) directs the Secretary of DHHS, acting through the Director of NIH, to establish a program for pediatric drug development. The Director of NIH delegated to the Director of NICHD, the authority and responsibility for establishment and conduct of that pediatric drug development activity as set forth in the legislation. The activities within BPCA for drug development fall into three general categories: identification of those drugs needing study, written requests from the FDA to the manufacturers to conduct pediatric studies deemed necessary for those drugs by the FDA, and if manufacturers declined to do these studies, referral of the drug to NIH to conduct the necessary testing.

In 2004 the NICHD began the third cycle of the annual process to develop a list of off-patent drugs prioritized for study under the provisions of the BPCA, and continues to closely coordinate its activities with other NIH Institutes/Centers and the Food and Drug Administration (FDA). During the last two years, NICHD has gained much experience from developing the 2003 and 2004 lists, as well as experience working with Written Requests (WRs) from the FDA.

Funding for the BPCA

In FY 2003, the NICHD identified $1.5 million in its budget to begin implementation of the BPCA. These funds provided the support to initiate a five-year contract for the BPCA Data Coordinating Center. For FYs 2004, 2005 and 2006 the NIH Director allocated $25.0 million each year from the budgets of the individual NIH Institutes and Center involved in pediatric research to continue implementation efforts.

In FY 2004, the $25.0 million was obligated as follows: $5.0 million for the Data Coordinating Center; $1.8 million for logistical support; $3.4 million for literature reviews; and approximately $14.8 million to initiate six drug studies. These obligations along with the total estimated costs over the life of the projects supported are included in Table 1 at the end of this report.

Studies Initiated During FY 2004

The list of off-patent priority drugs from which studies were initiated in FY 2004, under the Research Fund, was posted in a Federal Register Notice of February 2003. These six drugs, along with their indication for usage in pediatric populations, the estimated cost, and the current status of clinical testing can be found at the end of this report in Table 2. Criteria for selection included the frequency of use and overall public health impact.

Over the last year, the NICHD established mechanisms to gather existing information that supports the safe use of drugs in children and the types of conditions experienced in children that require pharmacotherapy. The NICHD awarded a series of contracts to gather information concerning pediatric conditions including: data on morbidity and hospitalizations in pediatric populations relating to frequency of outpatient medication use; analysis of Maryland Medicaid outpatient data; and analysis of inpatient frequency-of-use data. Contractors were asked to conduct systematic literature reviews and meta-analyses to provide summary information and assessments in support of the BPCA.

Drug Development Process

The drug development process needed to understand safety and efficacy for use in pediatric populations is complex, and generally, consists of preclinical and clinical phases. During the preclinical testing stage, the drug is tested for safety and efficacy in laboratory and animal studies. In general, preclinical studies involve pharmacology, toxicology, preformulation, formulation, analytical chemistry, and pharmacokinetics (which is the study of drug absorption, distribution, and elimination). An example of such a preclinical study being conducted by the NICHD, within the BPCA, is one involving a series of nonhuman primate studies to assess the scientific and safety concerns related to the use of Ketamine as an anesthetic in children. This study was initiated through an Intra-Agency Agreement (IAA) with the FDA.

During Phase I and II clinical studies, the drug is critically evaluated in humans to determine safety, while toxicology and pharmacokinetic testing continues. The purpose of this phase of testing is to assess the drug's mechanism of action in humans, pharmacokinetics, side effects of various doses, safe dosage range, and optimal route of administration.

Phase III studies, which expand the initial evaluations in humans, are closely controlled and generally conducted in several different clinical centers to determine the effectiveness of the drug for a particular indication in patients with the disease or condition under study. Participants in these studies are usually healthy except for the disease or condition being studied. There is usually a control and/or active agent comparison arm(s) in the study. The NICHD is presently conducting Phase I/II and Phase III clinical studies with Lorazepam (for sedation of children in an intensive care unit and for treatment of status epilepticus) and Nitroprusside (for acute control of blood pressure). Continued safety and additional efficacy parameters are evaluated during these clinical studies to determine ultimate labeling. Once a drug enters clinical trials in humans, it typically takes approximately five years for the trials to be completed and the FDA review finalized.

Collaborative Efforts Utilized to Initiate Drug Studies

During the last year, the NICHD has worked to strengthen its relationship with the FDA and other NIH Institutes. In addition, the NICHD has expanded its consultation with experts in pediatrics and pediatric pharmacology. The NICHD continues to work closely with the FDA in developing the Written Requests (WR) for off-patent drugs and clinical trial designs and in implementing both inpatient and outpatient pharmacotherapy. This collaboration between the NICHD and the FDA should lead to the development and implementation of clinical studies, which in turn should result in label modifications and improved pediatric therapeutics. Table 3 includes a list of drug studies being proposed for award during FY 2005.

In January 2004, the NICHD established a working group of FDA and NICHD staff to identify drugs for listing. In July 2004, the NICHD conducted its annual meeting with other NIH Institutes to discuss the status of FDA's WRs and to seek input regarding the 2005 List Process.

The NICHD also initiated a series of other activities in FY 2004 including:

- An agreement with the National Cancer Institute's (NCI) Children's Oncology Group (COG), to study the safety and efficacy of Vincristine and Dactinomycin for treatment of malignancies in children.
- An agreement with the FDA to conduct preclinical studies in non-human primates to evaluate the scientific and safety concerns about the use of Ketamine as an anesthetic in children.
- An agreement with the National Institute of Environmental Health Sciences (NIEHS) to acquire literature relating to the developmental and reproductive effects, general toxicity, and pharmacokinetics of Lindane (which is used on children to treat lice).
- A series of meetings with the National Institute of Mental Health (NIMH) to identify on-going pediatric clinical trials within the NIMH. Additionally, the NICHD is acquiring data sets created under an NIMH grant that will enhance information that the NICHD seeks to gather from a study of Lithium as it is used to treat bipolar disorder in the pediatric population.
- A contract with the Institute of Medicine (IOM) to identify and evaluate ethical issues concerning clinical trials in pediatric populations.
- Discussions with staff from the Office of Human Research Protection to implement the recommendations in the IOM report.

On-Patent Drugs

As of this writing, the FDA has referred the following five drugs and specific indications to the Foundation for the National Institutes of Health (FNIH) to consider for support of needed studies in children:

- Baclofen, for oral treatment of spasticity, most commonly from cerebral palsy
- Bupropion, for treatment of depression in children and smoking cessation in adolescents
- Sevelamer, to manage hyperphosphatemia in chronic renal insufficiency
- Morphine, for treatment of pain
- Zonisamide, for treatment of partial seizures

It is anticipated that the study of Baclofen will be initiated this fiscal year.

The List Development Process – FY 2004

The BPCA requires that the NIH annually identify the drugs of highest priority for study in pediatric populations. Initially, in June 2002, a drug prioritization process was established that attempted to rank each off-patent drug on the candidate list by considering use and potential public health benefit, and by combining this information with expert opinion and public discussion. Our experience with the initial process showed that much more information is needed about medications used with children, and the conditions for which the medications are used. As a result, the NICHD recognized the need to be adaptive and flexible in its approach to modifying the list in the coming years, as our knowledge grows about prescription medication use in children.

However, just based on the knowledge gained over the past two years, the NICHD identified three main areas for improvement. These include the following:

1) Creation of a more complete written record of the prioritization process;
2) Improvement of public access to the process as well as drawing on a wider range of expertise; and
3) Expansion of the knowledge base informing the process.

During the first two cycles of the list development process, informal efforts were made to consult with a variety of experts. Since then, the NICHD has implemented procedures that allow the Institute to take the process further by expanding the number of organizations contacted, and by widening the window of time within which we receive comments, input, and suggestions. The Institute also strove to increase public awareness of the list development process, and to increase opportunities for information sharing and discussion. To this end, the NICHD:

1) Shifted the time period of list development, so that preliminary lists were circulated widely in advance of publication in the Federal Register;
2) Developed an extensive list of organizations (medical, pediatric, nursing, pharmaceutical, and others) to receive information about the process and to solicit input;
3) Published a preliminary list in a <u>Federal Register</u> in August 2004 to solicit public comment; and
4) Held a scientific meeting several months in advance of publication of the list in a <u>Federal Register</u> to solicit comments and information.

Preparing the Priority List for January 2005

Since the enactment of the BPCA in January of 2002, the NICHD and the FDA have developed three lists of off-patent drugs that are candidates for further study in pediatric populations. Some minor additions and deletions have taken place such as some drugs coming off patent and, occasionally, some drugs going back on patent (i.e. if they are re-formulated). In April 2004, the list consisted of 206 off-patent or imminently off-patent drugs. This included the drugs prioritized in the 2003 lists, and the drugs eventually included in the 2004 lists. An additional 19 off-patent oncology drugs were added to the list in fall of 2004 resulting in a list of 225 off-patent drugs. In prioritizing drugs for 2005, the NICHD first excluded drugs from consideration that were already prioritized for study under the BPCA. After excluding these, the list consisted of 200 drugs.

To ensure the widest public health benefit, the NICHD incorporated data regarding frequency of use by children and the indications for such use. The NICHD is currently undertaking several initiatives to access and synthesize available data on frequency of use and to foster data collection where it is needed. The first efforts have yielded information regarding prescription medications used by an outpatient population covered by commercial insurance. In future years, the NICHD intends to incorporate data from Medicaid and other outpatient populations as well as data regarding inpatient medication use.

The NICHD obtained frequencies of medication use from Express Scripts, a pharmacy-benefits management company. Their database includes claims from individuals covered continuously or for part of the year; however, in this first analysis, data were included only if the person was enrolled for the entire year. The database is drawn from 30 million covered members in all 50 states during the year 2002. The analysis was restricted to children under age 18 and a total of

380,331 children were included. This initial analysis allowed the Institute to estimate the proportion of children using each drug, and then apply these estimates to the list of 200 drugs under consideration. Further analyses and publications reporting specifics of the analyses are being prepared; however, a striking feature of the results already is the wide variation in the frequency of use. Few off-patent drugs are used by more than 10 percent of all insured children in a given year: the sole exception is amoxicillin. A number of medications are used by less than 1/10,000 insured children in the same population and time period. Examples of this include acebutolol, oxazepam and triamterene. The NICHD decided to group medications by order of magnitude of use from 1/10 through 1/1,000,000 and ranked each medication accordingly.

Approximately 64 drugs were ranked as relatively high frequency, 39 drugs were ranked as relatively low frequency, and 97 drugs remained unranked because frequency data were not available. At least three reasons may explain the lack of information on frequency of use data: 1) either the drug is not used in an outpatient setting but used in an inpatient setting, 2) the drug is used in an outpatient setting but at extremely low frequency or not in the commercially insured population, and 3) the drug is not used by children in the United States. Until we explore these issues further, we are focusing attention on the 64 drugs ranked as relatively high frequency.

Need to Expand Knowledge Base

In developing the priority list of off-patent drugs, as called for under the BPCA, the NICHD strives to consider whether additional information is needed, whether new pediatric studies will produce health benefits, and whether reformulation of the drug is necessary.

In working with the FDA to prepare WRs for off-patent drugs, the NICHD noticed a paucity of sound data regarding medications and the frequency of their use by children and even less data describing indications for use. This issue arose while attempting to write WRs, as well as in translating WRs into Requests for Contracts. In both situations, data about frequency of use and indication for use would greatly facilitate design of studies and identification of key scientific questions. Therefore, the NICHD is striving to identify and solicit information about data sources and to promote analyses of available databases. Based on our efforts in 2004, the NICHD anticipates an influx of information beginning this year that will greatly aid the development of lists for 2006 and 2007. For this reason, the NICHD plans to revise the process each year, as it acquires useful information, and as it learns more about the use of prescription medications in children. This will require the NICHD to simplify the list development process to some degree and design the process with increased flexibility to incorporate new information.

The list process during FY 2004 culminated in a two-day scientific meeting that was held October 25 and 26, in Bethesda, Maryland. A committee of experts reviewed the semi-final draft list, and additionally, the NICHD solicited opinions and invited comments from interested parties. The meeting was open to the public and the proceedings were transcribed so they can be available for the public record. After the October meeting, the NICHD and the FDA finalized a list of 12 drugs that, after review within the NIH and the DHHS, were submitted to the Federal Register for publication in January 2005 (Tables 4 & 5).

The NICHD will continue to emphasize three factors (frequency of use, severity of the condition being treated, and potential for providing a public health benefit) in identifying drugs for study. However, the Institute also recognizes the need for more accurate and reliable estimates of frequency of use and comprehensive data regarding the frequency and severity of conditions before it can fully apply these factors in the decision process. Additionally, the NICHD recognizes the need for operational tools to rank severity, public health benefit, and other similar values in an objective and reproducible manner.

Conclusion

The NICHD is working closely with other Institutes and Centers within the NIH and with the FDA to identify off patent drugs that, if studied in children, would benefit pediatric therapeutics. In identifying those drugs, the NICHD is developing data resources that describe the frequency with which medications are used to treat children as well as the types of conditions experienced by children that bring them to practitioners. In developing the listing of drugs to be published in January 2005, the NICHD has provided more information on those that would benefit from clinical studies and those that should have systematic literature reviews based on expert input and comprehensive literature analysis.

Over the last three years that the NICHD has been implementing the BPCA, strong and coordinated collaboration with other IC's and the FDA has been established, and the Institute has reached out to pediatric experts and to others for input and advice. Pre-clinical and clinical studies have been initiated through contracts and interagency agreements for eight drug/indication pairs. These studies include literature analysis, preclinical animal studies as well as clinical trials. Much progress has been accomplished towards achieving the goal of safe drugs for children. However, due to the time required to complete pediatric studies and submit data to the FDA, it will take several years before labeling changes are implemented

---

Table 1: Projects Funded to Date with Yearly and Estimated Total Costs Through FY 2008
(Dollars in millions)

	FY 2003 Obligations	FY 2004 Obligations	Estimated Total Costs
Data Coordinating Center	$1.5	$5.0	$14.5
Drug Studies (see Table 2)	0	14.8	29.2
Literature Reviews	0	3.4	13.0
Logistical Support (includes workshops, conferences, professional support, IT support)	0	1.8	2.0
Total	1.5	25.0	$58.7

Table 2: Drug Studies Initiated During FY 2004
(Dollars in millions)

Performer/ Contractor	Drug/Indication	Type of Study	FY 2004 Obligations	Total Contract Costs	Anticipated date of study completion
Children's National Medical Center	Lorazepam - Treatment for status epilepticus	Pharmaco-kinetics (PK) Study	$1.6	$6.1	09/30/2008
Case Western	Lorazepam - Sedation of children on respirators in an intensive care unit	Randomized double-blind active comparator	4.8	9.0	03/31/2008
Duke	Nitroprusside - Control of blood pressure	Randomized double-blind parallel group	4.4	5.1	09/29/2007
Stanford	Nitroprusside - Control of blood pressure	Randomized double-blind parallel group	2.4	4.3	09/29/2007
National Cancer Institute's (NCI) Children's Oncology Group (COG)	Vincristine and Dactinomycin - Safety and efficacy of treatment for malignancies in children	Data gathering e.g., dose, efficacy, toxicity; age; diagnosis; planned PK study	1.3	3.7	2/28/2007
FDA	Ketamine - Preclinical studies in primates to evaluate the scientific and safety concerns about the use as an anesthetic in children	Preclinical studies	.3	1.0	09/30/2008
Total			14.8	29.2	

Table 3: Drug Studies Proposed for FY 2005

Drug	Indication	Estimated Cost For FY 2005	Status of Studies
Azithromycin	Ureaplasma pneumonia and BronchoPulmonaryDysplasia	$1.3	RFP Posted in Federal Business Opportunities
Azithromycin	Untreated maternal Chlamydia infection	1.0	RFP being issued
Meropenem	Complex pediatric abdominal infections	1.3	RFP being issued
Baclofen (On-Patent)	Oral treatment of spasticity, most commonly from cerebral palsy	2.1	RFP being issued
Lithium	Bipolar disorder in adolescents	1.0	RFP Posted in Federal Business Opportunities

Table 4: Drugs Reviewed at the 2004 Scientific Meeting and Recommended for Inclusion on the 2005 List

Drug	Patent Status	Indication
Ivermectin	Off-Patent	Scabies
Hydrocortisone Valerate ointment and cream	Off-Patent	Dermatitis
Hydrochlorothiazide	Off-Patent	Hypertension
Ethambutol	Off-Patent	Tuberculosis
Griseofulvin	Off-Patent	Tinea capitis
Methadone	Off-Patent	Opiate addicted neonates
Hydroxychloroquine	Off-Patent	Connective tissue disorders

Table 5: Status of Remaining Drugs for the 2005 Priority Listing

Drugs	Status	Indication	Recommendation
Acyclovir	Off-patent	Herpetic infections	Recommended for systematic literature review for potential re-labeling based on evidence available in the literature
Cyclosporine	Off-patent	Heart transplant patients	Recommended for systematic literature review and/or further consultation with scientific community to finalize scientific questions in need of study
Clonidine	Off-patent	Autism, attention deficit disorder	Recommended for systematic literature review and/or further consultation with scientific community to finalize scientific questions in need of study
Flecainide	Off-patent	Life threatening ventricular arrhythmias	Recommended for systematic literature review and/or further consultation with scientific community to finalize scientific questions in need of study
Bupropion	On-Patent	Depression	Recommended for systematic literature review and/or further consultation with scientific community

Mr. DEAL. The gentleman's time has expired. Ms. Blackburn.

Ms. BLACKBURN. Thank you, Dr. Zerhouni. If you get down to me, you know you are getting pretty close to the end. I am the only one left over here.

Just a couple of quick things, and you—Mr. Ferguson and Mr. Buyer both talked a little bit about your organization, and you mentioned where you would have put some focus this year if you had had funding. But I want to go back to something that Dr. Varmus, who was your predecessor, had said in 2001. He mentioned that he felt like you could add 10 Institutes a decade, and what I am hearing from you is you probably would opt not to that—not to do that, but would work within your framework, and use the flexibility from the proposed legislation to allow you to meet those needs. Is that a correct understanding?

Mr. ZERHOUNI. Right. I know Dr. Varmus well, and what he was referring to, what he told me, is that unless we have a mechanism to prevent proliferation, we will end up with 10 per decade, and then make the agency less manageable. He has advocated, actually, consolidation of all Institutes into five Institutes. So he is clearly one who has been very concerned about the rapid growth of the number of Institutes.

Ms. BLACKBURN. Excellent, and thank you for the clarification on that. A little bit on flexibility and collaboration, and let me use, to make the point, use the SARS outbreak, because I have read that you all did some research and some work on SARS in 2003. Now, we are hearing about avian flu, and the possibility of avian flu. So using SARS as our real life example, and our experience, talk to me just a little bit about how quickly you were able to put funding into the Institute for Allergy and Infectious Diseases, and the old structure, what your turnaround was on meeting the need for research, and then, the new structure, how you would plan to do that, and if St. Jude's, which is right in Shelby County, which— one of the counties I represent—is doing some avian flu work. So how quickly would the new legislation allow you to respond, and how would it make it easier than the old legislation?

Mr. ZERHOUNI. Very important points. In the SARS case, we had invested NIAID, the National Institute of Allergy and Infectious Diseases, invested in Asia years ago, in having laboratories in Asia, to, in fact, be our sort of warning stations for flu. We actually thought it was flu at the beginning. When we identified, CDC identified that this was a different disease, we then collaborated with CDC, and very quickly, were able to identify the virus. Now, you are asking what did you then do to develop a vaccine to—for SARS? The Institute then reallocated resources, because of the doubling, we have built a Vaccine Research Center, which is extremely capable, so that the fundamental investment was there, and then the Director of the Institute reallocated dollars within its Institute to develop the early prototypes of two, and now, three SARS vaccines, one of which is in trial.

In the case of pandemic flu, this is a much larger problem. The Secretary Levitt has appointed a taskforce that is being coordinated across the government. There is no doubt that we need to be able to move resources. In the current context, it is not that easy to do. I can use transfer authority if I need to. It is 1 percent of that. We can also, obviously, use a 1 percent transfer authority the Secretary has, to be able to move dollars in that category. You can use contracts. So in the case of flu, we have been able—over a year ago, we knew that there was a risk of flu, to develop a prototype vaccine, and we have a prototype vaccine. We have 2 million doses, and it has been tested last—this past few months.

Ms. BLACKBURN. And under your existing structure, how quickly were you able to do that, and under the proposed structure, how quickly would you anticipate being able to do that?

Mr. ZERHOUNI. The current structure that is being proposed is really to be more strategic and proactive in known public health problems——

Ms. BLACKBURN. Okay. So it would not affect that. One quick thing, one last question. I like your mission statement, and basically, what it is saying is science in pursuit of knowledge to improve health. So as you look at your mission, and we talk about the proposed legislation, does the legislation improve your ability to meet your mission?

Mr. ZERHOUNI. I believe so. I think improvements in our ability to coordinate and synergize the 27 Institutes and Centers is very important to science today. If you look at the key elements of science today, one, it has become interdisciplinary. You need people from physical sciences, computer science, mathematics, working with biologists. So they cannot be locked into silos.

Second, the scale of experiments that we do is larger, and there is—and when I started research, we had three members of my team, myself and two co-investigators. You go to any scientific meeting today, or look at a publication in any journal, you will have 15 collaborators. So collaboration is very important as well. This means that Institutes and NIH in general needs to be more nimble and more aggressive in stimulating and incubating these sorts of approaches, and I think it will do that.

Ms. BLACKBURN. Thank you.

Mr. DEAL. Ms. Capps.

Ms. CAPPS. Thank you, Mr. Chairman, and Dr. Zerhouni, thank you very much for spending this entire afternoon here with us. I appreciate your testimony.

In it, you referred several times to the report of the Institute of Medicine, and I want to refer to the Institute's recommendation No. 4, regarding the ability to respond to new challenges, for enhancing and increasing trans-NIH strategic planning, the D part of that, which designates, or they recommend a percentage of each Institute to be preserved for trans-NIH research. Today, in your testimony, you have spoken several times, and have referred in some of your responses to questions about a common fund for trans-NIH research. I would like to give you the opportunity to spell out what you mean. Do you see this as a standalone pot of money, or is it sufficient to require, as the IOM suggests, and just elaborate as to how you talk about that common fund?

Mr. ZERHOUNI. So effectively, you can handle it in, like I said, in three different ways. I think what the IOM is recommending is what I call the common fund.

Ms. CAPPS. Right.

Mr. ZERHOUNI. So in other words, you know that 5 percent of your budget is going to be not determined by you, as NIH Institute—I mean, as, by an Institute Director, but it will be put in a common pool, to be jointly planned, jointly decided for, initiatives that are important, emerging, and so on. That is the common fund concept.

Ms. CAPPS. I understand. Now, that is part of the—each Institute's budget.

Mr. ZERHOUNI. It is part of the mission——

Ms. CAPPS. That they are going to set aside for that.

Mr. ZERHOUNI. Yes. I don't think it is necessary, No. 1, to take away from the Institutes.

Ms. CAPPS. Right.

Mr. ZERHOUNI. In their base. Second, I don't think it is necessary for the Director to have grant-making authority. I think—I don't think you need to be grant making. You don't want to create an Institute——

Ms. CAPPS. That is what I wanted to really be clear about.

Mr. ZERHOUNI. Right.

Ms. CAPPS. Do you want the Office of the Director, whether it is you or whoever it is, to have direct grant making authority?

Mr. ZERHOUNI. No. I think grant coordination, resource allocation decision, planning authorities, to be able to look across and not be told, well, this is not really your money, it is my money.

Ms. CAPPS. Right. So but you——

Mr. ZERHOUNI. That phenomenon needs to go away.

Ms. CAPPS. But what role would you play, or the Director play, in this?

Mr. ZERHOUNI. Coordination.

Ms. CAPPS. Just coordination.

Mr. ZERHOUNI. Yes, strategic coordination, just what it says, program coordination across the silos, strategic initiatives, create a transparent process, that is based on an analytical framework that is good for analysis, good reporting.

Ms. CAPPS. Okay.

Mr. ZERHOUNI. This is just basically decision support——

Ms. CAPPS. Okay.

Mr. ZERHOUNI. [continuing] mechanism. Not take the money away, not—nor become, in—a twenty-eighth Institute. I don't think——

Ms. CAPPS. Right.

Mr. ZERHOUNI. I don't think that is a good idea.

Ms. CAPPS. I see. It—and do you have ideas about—is it a permanent set aside of this funding mechanism, or——

Mr. ZERHOUNI. If you don't make it permanent, you will never change the culture. They don't——

Ms. CAPPS. So you are using this as a way of changing the culture, getting at your ideas of responsibility——

Mr. ZERHOUNI. Of the margins, yes, to instill the fact, and the need to coordinate better for scientific challenges that have become bigger and larger.

Ms. CAPPS. So I want—I am going to turn to another topic, but I wanted to make sure—this is something that you really have pulled out of the Institute of Medicine report, and you really want to see that as a focus of the new NIH, as your envisioning it——

Mr. ZERHOUNI. Right.

Ms. CAPPS. [continuing] as being more flexible.

Mr. ZERHOUNI. Well, from my standpoint on the IOM report, this recommendation No. 4 is critical.

Ms. CAPPS. All right.

Mr. ZERHOUNI. And I support it.

Ms. CAPPS. Okay. Great. Another topic, since I have a little bit of time left, there—in the draft legislation that the committee is preparing, there is a new division, the Division of Program Coordination, Planning, and Strategic Initiatives, to oversee and coordinate the offices currently located within the Office of Director, and so forth. In other words, in a way, you could say a new bureaucracy, but I, you know, I don't want to cast a negative word on that.

I have heard some concern that creating a new division to carry out these functions could weaken the authority of the existing Office. It could make for more reporting, when you are talking about that there is already a lot, and—so can you comment on what you see as the ideal model for managing coordination and strategic planning at NIH, since this is such an important focus for the future?

Mr. ZERHOUNI. Again, I don't think that division should be in charge of all strategic planning for all missions at NIH.

Ms. CAPPS. Okay.

Mr. ZERHOUNI. That should be left to the Institutes. It is really the synchronization and coordination that this division should be doing. As far as the Offices, remember, the Offices were created because there was somewhere, somehow, a need, felt by many people in the community, including Congress, for better coordination.

Ms. CAPPS. Okay.

Mr. ZERHOUNI. That is why they were created in law. So I think they should continue their role. They should be coordinated, but the problem that you are talking about, bureaucracy, is every time you create a new structure——

Ms. CAPPS. Yes.

Mr. ZERHOUNI. [continuing] you have created a new bureaucracy, and that is what I think we need to avoid. We need to find ways of preserving their role and continue their mission. I mean, the Office of AIDS Research plays a very important role.

Ms. CAPPS. Right.

Mr. ZERHOUNI. Look at the authorities of that office.

Ms. CAPPS. Right.

Mr. ZERHOUNI. I mean, OAR looks at the AIDS budget across NIH. That should be continued.

Ms. CAPPS. Just to be clear, and kind of as a way of giving us advice on designing this legislation, would existing Offices need to report to the division? Is there a chain of command here?

Mr. ZERHOUNI. Well, I think the division should be pulling from their staff, division of the Director. So to me, the Director should really take a role here, because he or she is accountable. The problem is, if she is accountable, shows up at hearings like this——

Ms. CAPPS. I see.

Mr. ZERHOUNI. [continuing] when there is a problem, but they don't necessarily have the authority to be able to be accountable, so I think the divisions should be part of the Office of the Director.

Ms. CAPPS. And when you say coordinator, you give a lot of authority to coordinator. I mean, that is—you are saying that is where your responsibility lies, or the Director's responsibility.

Mr. ZERHOUNI. That is right. Yes, over a——

Ms. CAPPS. Kind of a bottom line.

Mr. ZERHOUNI. Well, that is—portion of the budget that should be jointly planned and jointly executed.

Ms. CAPPS. Thank you, Dr. Zerhouni.

Mr. ZERHOUNI. Thank you.

Mr. DEAL. Mr. Green.

Mr. GREEN. Thank you, Mr. Chairman. I ask unanimous consent to have a statement placed in the record.

Dr. Zerhouni, the current organization at NIH affords the Institute in Cancer, and Center Directors, with a great amount of autonomy in priority setting, Director of the National Cancer Institute is arguably an even greater autonomy, since he has the ability to take the NCI budget directly to the OMB. This structure has enabled cancer research to develop new therapies, and to make great strides toward cancer. Under the organization structure proposed in this draft legislation, would have the NIH Director have sole responsibility for priority setting. While the draft remains silent on budgetary bypass authority for NCI, do you envision the NCI retaining that authority to go directly to the OMB?

Mr. ZERHOUNI. First of all, the NIH Director should have the sole priority setting authority. I hope I made myself clear, Mr. Chairman and Mr. Green, that it needs to be balanced. It needs to be part of a coordinating effort that should not be subject to the veto of every 27 Institutes and Centers. That is what I mean by the reason to do that, but beyond that percentage of trans-NIH initiatives, I think the Institutes should retain their fundamental missions and authorities, and in the case of the National Cancer Institute, I think it has been very important to the NCI, and to its community, from what I hear, this authority to go and have a bypass budget and so on is critical to their mission. So I think it should be preserved, provided that they also participate in the common fund for the common good.

Mr. GREEN. The draft legislation strikes a number of authorizations that are either expired or never been appropriated. It is clear from the intent that the bill is to strike expired authorizations of appropriations, while maintaining authority to carry out these programs. I am interested how the NIH views these authorizations in setting priorities. For instance, in 2000, Congress passed the Clinical Research Enhancement Act, which included a clinical research loan repayment program, to encourage investigators with medical school debt to pursue a career in clinical research. However, during the Congressional consideration of that legislation, NIH made clear to us that the loan repayment program needed specific authorization in order to make the program available to extramural researchers—NIH campus. Would the strikes contained in this bill lead you to discontinue the Clinical Research Loan Program, and can you speak to the overall impact, if any, on these strikes to the NIH continuing the Clinical Research Program?

Mr. ZERHOUNI. That is a good question. I really—this is obviously a technical issue. I am not clear about the authorities that we have, but I do know that we do have the authority to do loan repayment in PHS, authority, as I testified. I would—definitely would like to have my legal people help me with that, and get back to you on the record.

[The following was received for the record:]

Removal of the "authorization of appropriation" provisions would not affect the NIH's ability to conduct clinical research programs, including loan repayment programs, authorized by statute, so long as appropriations are deemed available. The changes and additions to the authorizing legislation to enable extramural clinical researchers to apply for loan repayment made by the Clinical Research Enhancement Act were necessary because prior NIH statutory authority only provided for a loan repayment program for clinical researchers from disadvantaged backgrounds who agreed to conduct clinical research as employees of the NIH.

Mr. GREEN. Well, the biggest concern I have about that is their impact on the goal of attracting health professionals to careers in clinical research.

Mr. ZERHOUNI. Absolutely. I understand very well.

Mr. GREEN. And my last question, Mr. Chairman, the bill contains four broad authorization levels, that authorize appropriation for individual Institutes or Centers. If this draft bill were to become law, and the Appropriations Committee continued to provide line item appropriations for individual Centers and Institutes, would—the result would essentially be unauthorized appropriations. Of course, this scenario happens quite frequently here in Congress, that we have approved money, but appropriation for money that is not authorized. Is it your preference to receive four different appropriated amounts, or would you prefer that Congress provide individual Institutes and Centers with line item appropriations, and can you speak to that role, that increased transfer authority plays in that scenario? For example, I know you talked about the certain percentage in—for example, if NIH were to receive appropriations that mirror these four authorization groups, why is it individual transfer necessary? You are already deviating, or divvying up the money individually.

Mr. ZERHOUNI. As I mentioned in my previous, I think it is very—from my standpoint and my experience, I think it is extremely important that whatever we do, we do it progressively, and whatever happens, we can't overnight make wholesale changes at NIH. It is not possible. So whatever the committee eventually decides to do, we need to retain the ability to maintain the momentum, and whatever I am talking about, in terms of transfer authorities, or common fund, or opportunity, however it settles, we need to really, also, make sure that there is a smooth transition from State A to State B. And I guess I am being—I am answering both questions at once.

Mr. GREEN. Yes.

Mr. ZERHOUNI. There is value to making sure that this goes to that mission, for that amount, and that it doesn't change erratically from year to year, because we have to maintain these programs over time, and second, I think it is important to understand the difference between a transfer authority which is post facto, a common fund, which is prospective, an opportunity fund, which is responsive to—and this is where I think we need to have more interactions with the committee, which I think we have had, and refine that concept.

Mr. GREEN. Mr. Chairman, since my time has run out, and I just appreciate, Dr. Zerhouni, for your patience this afternoon. Obviously, there is a lot of interest on both sides of the aisle, because so many of us are proud of what NIH is doing with all the Institutes, although I understand the organizational chart can be a nightmare. We just don't want to lose all the success we have had.

Thank you, Mr. Chairman.

Mr. DEAL. Thank the gentleman. Mr. Engel.

Mr. ENGEL. Thank you. Thank you, Mr. Chairman, Dr. Zerhouni. I saw, I listened to your presentation, your testimony, and the slideshow, and I have to say that you make a very good case for the need for change.

I have two specific questions regarding that that I would like to ask, but I do think that the slides and your presentation were on the money. I mean, some of us have some questions about some of the nuances, but I think overall, I think the vision is a good one.

I want to talk to you first about the Office of AIDS Research. That has been very much praised as a model for strategic planning for many years, and for budgeting, because the OAR has the statutory authority and responsibility to develop a comprehensive strategic plan, with input from the NIH ICs, and from nongovernmental scientists, and community advocates, and everyone involved with AIDS. The OAR director has the authority to move resources across the different Institutes to address scientific priorities that may change from year to year, and the draft bill, I think, and correct me if I am wrong, implies that the NIH Director would now, and I have a quote, "be responsible for strategic planning and priority setting of all research activities conducted or supported by the NIH." That is the quote. Lots of people have expressed concern to me that the expanded authority of the NIH Director could undermine the existing statutory authorities of the Office of AIDS Research provided by Congress, and I am wondering if you could comment on that.

Mr. ZERHOUNI. A very good question. I think there is a tremendous amount, sometimes, of anxiety about any change, so you can hear, but I think we need to be responsive to that. First of all, I consider the model at OAR has been a good model. Think about it. The Director of NIH never had that authority over any part of the portfolio of NIH. Yet, OAR has it. OAR can look strategically, get counsel from the Institutes, look at the portfolio, reassign the portfolio. Like, for example, Dr. Jack Whitescarver changed the priority to vaccines over the past 2 years, because we have now vaccines candidates we want to try. It is changed to what drugs, at the time; that was progressive. Likewise, I think it is understandable, and I think the committee is sort of paralleling my own thoughts, and the thoughts of the IOM and others, to say why wouldn't the Director of NIH also have that same sort of OAR type authority over a common fund—what is wrong with that—without taking away from the important mission of OAR?

So my view is that these are complementary, not exclusionary of each other. I think the NIH Director needs to have what I would call generic authority over a small portion of the budget, just like OAR has specific authority over 10 percent of the NIH budget, which is the AIDS portfolio.

Mr. ENGEL. But you can certainly understand why there would be some transition.

Mr. ZERHOUNI. Absolutely. Absolutely, and I believe that, as I said in my slideshow, that those Institutes should retain their role—I mean those Offices.

Mr. ENGEL. Thank you. My second question is about translational research. It has been a major priority, obviously, of the NIH, and I have a very specific question. How would the legislation affect the agency's ability to promote and conduct translational research, especially in areas such as research on Charcot-Marie-Tooth Disorder, which has the potential to translate into direct benefits for other—research into other neurodegenerative disorders, such as ALS and multiple sclerosis?

Mr. ZERHOUNI. I think that is a very interesting question, of what would happen, if the only way this structure will change, if Charcot-Marie-Tooth is obviously a disease that we are responsible for, and we have a mission to help. But let us suppose something new happened in either the therapeutic world, or—and something that no single Institute could put in place. That new structure would basically look at that, and potentially, allocate common resources for an emerging area of opportunity that would be relevant to that disease, but this structure is not dedicated or designed to serve special purpose outcomes. Diseases, organs, life stages, cross cutting science, should be primarily done in its great majority by the Institutes in their missions as specified. The structure should only be the glue for things that are of common interest to all. So it may not be relevant to a specific disease, but it could be relevant to something that is emerging, that is affecting the landscape of science in one way that may be relevant to Charcot-Marie-Tooth for that particular case. So sometimes, for example, we have in trial right now a drug, to potentially be important for ALS. It is an antibiotic. No one knew that it could have a role. Well, reacting quickly to that would require, perhaps, a discussion, a coming together of all the Institutes, and say this is something novel, this is something we need to try. That might be impacted at that point.

Mr. ENGEL. Well, thank you, and let me just conclude by thanking you for staying this long, and thanking you for the great job you are doing. Thank you, sir.

Mr. ZERHOUNI. Thank you.

Mr. DEAL. Dr. Zerhouni, we likewise reiterate our appreciation for your being here today. I think you can tell the committee has great interest in what we are doing. By our accounts, some 29 members have spent at least some quality time with us this afternoon, and I appreciate your patience, and if you wish to supplement or add additional information for the record, you may certainly be free to do so.

I would like to also pay tribute to Cheryl Jaeger, who is our staff person primarily responsible for this major undertaking, and express our appreciation to her for her hard work, as we try to finalize this product, and to my colleague, Mr. Brown, for his patience as well.

There being nothing further to come before the committee, this hearing is adjourned.

Mr. ZERHOUNI. Thank you, Mr. Chairman.

[Whereupon, at 4:40 p.m., the committee was adjourned.]

[Additional material submitted for the record follows:]

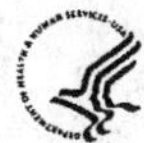

DEPARTMENT OF HEALTH & HUMAN SERVICES   Public Health Service

National Institutes of Health
Bethesda, Maryland 20892

NOV 0 8 2005

The Honorable Nathan Deal
Chairman, House Energy and Commerce
 Subcommittee on Health
United States House of Representatives
Washington, D.C. 20515

Dear Chairman Deal:

I am responding to your September 15, 2005, letter to Dr. Elias Zerhouni, Director of the National Institutes of Health (NIH), following up on the July 19, 2005, hearing entitled: "Legislation to Reauthorize the National Institutes of Health." Enclosed are responses to the questions you forwarded from members of the House Committee on Energy and Commerce. We look forward to working with the Committee as it works to reauthorize NIH.

I have also provided a copy of this response to Representatives Barton, Brown, DeGette, Markey and Waxman.

Sincerely,

Marc Smolonsky
Associate Director for
 Legislative Policy and Analysis

Enclosures

<u>Question from the Honorable Diana DeGette</u>
Dr. Elias Zerhouni, Director
National Institutes of Health
July 19, 2005
Committee on Energy and Commerce hearing entitled, "Legislation to Reauthorize the National Institutes of Health"

1. What is the NIH doing to prepare for/prevent a global pandemic of the avian flu? Do you have a strategy in place to prepare for such a possibility? Are there adequate resources at this time?

> The Department of Health and Human Services (DHHS) has developed a Draft Pandemic Influenza Preparedness and Response Plan, which outlines a coordinated national strategy to prepare for and respond to an influenza pandemic. The Plan assigns specific roles to several Federal agencies; the National Institute of Allergy and Infectious Diseases (NIAID) holds the primary responsibility for carrying out those duties assigned to the NIH.

> Specifically, the role of the NIAID is to conduct basic research and to develop and clinically evaluate new medical interventions -- vaccines, antivirals and diagnostics -- that may lead to more effective approaches to controlling influenza virus infections. These activities provide a critical research foundation for influenza preparedness and complement the roles of the Centers for Disease Control and Prevention (CDC) and the Food and Drug Administration (FDA).

> NIAID's multi-faceted approach to address the threat of avian influenza includes vaccine and antiviral development as well as surveillance, basic research, and genome sequencing. Specific examples of research and development activities conducted or supported by NIAID are listed below.

> **Vaccine Development - H5N1 Influenza**
> - NIAID awarded a contract for the manufacturing and production of H5N1 inactivated vaccine in May 2004 to Aventis (sanofi) pasteur, and sanofi pasteur delivered the vaccine to NIAID in early March 2005. NIAID's Vaccine and Treatment Evaluation Units (VTEUs) currently are conducting a clinical trial using the sanofi pasteur vaccine in healthy adults. Preliminary data in a subset of participants indicated that the vaccine is generally safe and able to stimulate an immune response. Future plans include testing the sanofi pasteur H5N1 vaccine in elderly and pediatric populations.
> - NIAID also awarded a contract for the manufacture and production of H5N1 inactivated vaccine to Chiron in May 2004. The Chiron vaccine is expected to be provided to NIAID for evaluation in clinical trials by the end of 2005.
> - NIAID intramural researchers have developed three live attenuated H5N1 cold-adapted vaccine candidates, which have been shown to be protective in mice. The researchers will work with colleagues from MedImmune, Inc., under a Cooperative Research and Development Agreement to produce and test multiple

vaccine candidates for potential pandemic flu strains, including H5N1 strains. Future plans include generating clinical lots of vaccine and conducting clinical trials. The vaccines would be administered as a nasal spray.

Vaccine Development - H9N2 Influenza
- Under contract to NIAID, Chiron produced an H9N2 inactivated vaccine. A Phase I clinical trial in healthy adults started in March 2005.
- NIAID intramural scientists developed an H9N2 cold-adapted vaccine candidate. A clinical lot of this vaccine was generated and a Phase I clinical trial of the safety and immunogenicity of the vaccine for healthy adults has been undertaken.

Vaccine Development - Dose-Sparing Strategies
- NIAID has completed enrollment and vaccinated participants in a study to compare intramuscular vs. intradermal vaccination with the sanofi pasteur H5N1 vaccine. Data from this study are expected in late 2005.
- NIAID has trials of avian influenza vaccines with adjuvants (alum, MF59) planned for 2006, including trials of the sanofi pasteur and Chiron H5N1 vaccines and the Chiron H9N2 vaccine.

Antiviral Development
NIAID funded projects to develop improved antivirals include:
- Development and testing of a long-acting next-generation neuraminidase inhibitor[1] that can be administered once per week, which could help ease logistical burdens such as storage and distribution;
- Combination animal study to determine if administration of treatment with both a neuraminidase inhibitor and an adamantane is more effective than treatment with a single antiviral in reducing viral replication and emergence of drug resistant strains;
- Evaluation of novel drug targets for potential prevention and treatment of influenza using *in vitro* and animal models.

Surveillance - Animal Influenza in Asia
- Through a contract to St. Jude Children's Research Hospital, NIAID is funding disease surveillance in wild birds, live bird markets, and pigs in Hong Kong, which allows scientists to track potential emergent influenza strains.
- In January 2005, this contract was expanded to include animal surveillance in Vietnam, Thailand, and Indonesia.
- Researchers supported by the contract also are developing a variety of vaccine reference strains, including the H5N1 "seed strain" used to produce the sanofi pasteur H5N1 vaccine currently under investigation.

---

[1]The surfaces of influenza viruses are dotted with neuraminidase proteins. Neuraminidase, an enzyme, breaks the bonds that hold new virus particles to the outside of an infected cell. Once the enzyme breaks these bonds, this sets free new viruses that can infect other cells and spread infection. Neuraminidase inhibitors block the enzyme's activity and prevent new virus particles from being released, thereby limiting the spread of infection.

Basic and Applied Research

NIAID supports a number of basic and applied research projects that could lead to significant advances against avian influenza, including:

- Alternatives to using chicken eggs for vaccine production;
- Strategies for rapid production of a vaccine against a newly emergent virus strain;
- Vaccines that provide broad protection against multiple virus strains;
- Gene-based influenza vaccines;
- Research on virus structure and function, viral pathogenesis, and the host response to infection.

Influenza Genome Sequencing

NIAID is supporting a collaborative effort to release full genomic sequence information for several thousand influenza viruses to the public domain via the National Library of Medicine's National Center for Biotechnology information. More than 350 influenza viruses have been sequenced. Readily available sequence data will allow researchers to:

- Further study how influenza viruses evolve, spread, and cause disease, which may ultimately lead to improved methods of treatment and prevention;
- Identify specific characteristics of previous pandemic strains, which may help focus preparedness efforts;
- Identify genes that are highly conserved among various strains, and therefore may be good targets for broadly protective therapeutics or vaccines.

The NIAID has made significant progress with available resources in understanding the epidemiology and structure of pandemic influenza virus strains, in developing potential antivirals, and in assisting our industry partners in developing vaccine candidates. The NIAID continues to pursue this multi-pronged approach to fulfilling NIH's responsibilities under the Draft Pandemic Influenza Preparedness and Response Plan. The NIAID will continue to coordinate its activities with other Federal agencies to ensure preparedness for a possible influenza pandemic.

<u>**Questions from the Honorable Edward J. Markey**</u>
Dr. Elias Zerhouni, Director
National Institutes of Health
July 19, 2005
Committee on Energy and Commerce hearing entitled, "Legislation to Reauthorize the National Institutes of Health"

1. Currently, the Appropriations Committee provides a separate line item for each of the Institutes. If this bill passes, do you hope that the Appropriations Committee will continue appropriating in that way or do you hope that they will give lump sums to the two groups of Institutes and allow you to determine the levels of funding for the different Institutes within the groups?

    I believe that in order to preserve the momentum of the NIH Institutes and Centers (ICs) separate appropriations line items should continue.

2. If this bill passes, will you continue to ask Congress for separate appropriations for each of the different Institutes or will you just ask for one appropriation for the mission specific Institutes and another for the science enabling Institutes?

    I will continue to ask for separate appropriations for each IC.

3. Cancer advocates from my State are concerned that this bill may change the special status of the National Cancer Institute. How do you think this bill will change that special status?

    I believe the bill will not alter NCI's special authorities. More importantly, I recognize the central role that NCI plays in the fight against cancer and will continue to preserve the unique authorities currently given to the NCI Director.

4. Do you believe that creating a registry of clinical trials that would include the results of those trials would help secure the public trust in medical research and advances the goals of NIH?

    Yes, I believe that enhancing access to clinical trials and trial results will increase public trust in medical research and that enhanced access is in keeping with the goals of NIH's mission. Indeed, NIH has a long-standing commitment to ensuring broad access to knowledge gained through the efforts it funds. The NIH Director's Council of Public Representatives (COPR), as part of its deliberations on the issue of public participation and trust in research, recommended that study results and outcomes from NIH-funded research be shared with research participants and the larger community promptly and consistently.

    Achieving this goal will take time, but we are working now on the critical first step to this process which is ensuring that ClinicalTrials.gov includes links to peer-reviewed publications and result reports that are already in the public domain.

5. The National Library of Medicine currently runs a registry of clinical trials that is mandatory
    for trials that look at serious or life-threatening diseases. However, the registry does not have
    any enforcement mechanisms, so it is essentially a voluntary registry. Can you please tell me
    how industry compliance has been? Is the current database complete and accurate for serious
    and life-threatening diseases?

> An August 2005[2] report by FDA on the implementation of Section 113 of FDAMA
> provides some data on industry compliance with the law. The report indicates that
> industry compliance was 30 percent overall during a nine-month period in 2002. By
> comparison, during a three-month period in 2004, 70 percent of cancer trials were
> submitted. The FDA report concluded that while progress has been made in achieving
> better registration rates, further work is needed by all concerned parties to assure
> increased participation in ClinicalTrials.gov.
>
> Steps taken last year by the International Committee of Medical Journal Editors (ICMJE)
> may also be helpful. Representing 14 leading medical journals, ICMJE announced that,
> beginning in September 2004, it would require the registration of "clinically directive"
> trials at inception as a precondition for publication of manuscripts using the results.
> Although it is too early to know the long-term effect of the policy, there has been an
> increase in trial submissions to ClinicalTrials.gov since the ICMJE policy was instituted.
> Industry registered 1,981 studies (compared to 241 registrations from the same period in
> 2004) and universities, foundations, and other non-profit organizations registered 3,989
> studies (28 in 2004).

6. Dr. Zerhouni, some in the pharmaceutical industry and the research community have
    suggested that they could create a voluntary registry of clinical trials that would provide the
    public with complete and accurate information about drugs and medical devices. From your
    experience running what amounts to a voluntary registry, do you believe that it is possible for
    a voluntary registry without any enforcement mechanisms or any oversight to ensure the
    quality of the data to provide the public with complete and accurate information?

> There is strong and growing support in many quarters for national trial registration in a
> publicly accessible database, and I am hopeful that the efforts that are being made by
> public and private organizations will help us achieve this goal. As data from FDA's
> status report on the implementation of Section 113 indicates, industry compliance with
> ClinicalTrials.gov registration has been improving. Congressional and public interest
> certainly helps increase support for trial registration. For our part, we are exploring a
> number of ways of increasing registration and are taking steps to ensure that
> ClinicalTrials.gov can provide the platform for such a national registry.

7. The website, Clinicaltrials.gov, does not provide the results to clinical trials, yet you have
    said that it would be important for the medical community to have access to that information.
    Do you believe that Clinicaltrials.gov, which is run by the National Library of Medicine,
    could be expanded to include a results database?

---

[2] http://www.fda.gov/oashi/clinicaltrials/section113/113report/

We have been actively exploring this question for a number of months. An internal working group was established last fall to consider whether an expanded collection of information about the results of NIH-funded studies is necessary and feasible and, if so, how best to implement such a program. Based on the group's findings, we think that it will be possible for NIH to use ClinicalTrials.gov to enhance access to information about trial results, first by ensuring that all journal citations are added for published trials and then through the development of a standard data format for the display of results summaries (not the raw data itself) from both published and unpublished studies. That said, it is important to acknowledge the significant challenges associated with assembling summary information about results in the absence of peer scientific and editorial review, as well as the legal issues that must be addressed. As such, before implementing enhanced access through ClinicalTrials.gov, we will be undertaking a broad consultation within NIH and among all interested parties in the intramural and extramural communities and among patient groups, industry collaborators, foundations, and medical editors. These consultations will ensure that the full range of interests affected by enhanced access are taken into consideration.

8. Does NIH currently have the authority to require results of clinical trials?

The answer to the question of whether NIH has authority to require results of clinical trials, or the submission of clinical trial results to a national database, is complex. First, it is important to remember that NIH's authorities pertain to NIH employees and recipients of NIH funding, not to the private sector, e.g., the pharmaceutical industry, or other sponsors of research. In addition, while we may have authority to require grantees to provide progress reports and final study outcome summaries, implementing a requirement for the submission of results in a usable, standard format for posting to a national registry would require the promulgation of new policies and procedures that implicate, for example, requirements of the Administrative Procedures Act and Paperwork Reduction Act. In addition, grantees have intellectual property rights under the Bayh-Dole Act that would need to be considered. Consistent with applicable law, any new policy would need to allow grant recipients to seek patent protection as necessary for development of a research product. NIH would also need to provide grantees with sufficient time to publish results prior to posting on a publicly accessible database. These issues are very important and will be considered as part of our next broad consultation steps.

Questions from the Honorable Henry A. Waxman
Dr. Elias Zerhouni, Director
National Institutes of Health
July 19, 2005
Committee on Energy and Commerce hearing entitled, "Legislation to Reauthorize the National Institutes of Health"

There is general agreement that NIH should pursue more cross-cutting, interdisciplinary initiatives. An important question is how these can be financed. One option is to give the NIH Director the power to transfer large amounts of funding from institute to institute after the appropriations process.

1. Would large transfers after the appropriations process be disruptive to the work of scientists in NIH institutes?

    Yes.

2. Could planning by the institutes suffer if there were uncertainty about the availability of funding?

    Yes.

An alternative approach to promoting interdisciplinary initiatives is to establish "escrow" accounts at each institute. Each institute would set aside a certain percentage - such as 5% – of their budget for use in interdisciplinary research.

3. How would an "escrow account" approach help promote coordination of research at NIH?

    The "escrow account" to which you refer is what I call the "Common Fund" which would finance trans-NIH initiatives recommended by the proposed Division of Program Coordination, Planning, and Strategic Initiatives (DPCPSI). I envision the Common Fund as a set aside where an agreed upon percent of the budget of each Institute and Center (IC) is allocated for efforts identified by DPCPSI though a transparent planning process and according to defined criteria. Having the ICs vested in the Common Fund provides an incentive to the ICs to participate in trans-NIH activities.

4. Would an "escrow account" model allow for more stability and planning at the institutes than a possible significant loss of funding from transfers?

    The Common Fund should grow incrementally and be guided by NIH budget growth. I believe this model would provide stability and will allow the ICs to plan for their own research initiatives.

The Institute of Medicine recommended that the NIH fund more "high risk, high reward" research. To decide which research to fund, the IOM recommended that special peer review panels be constituted that can recognize promising proposals that otherwise might have been rejected as too speculative.

However, the idea has also been floated that the NIH Director should be able to fund these projects without peer review and absent standard protections against waste, fraud, and abuse.

5. Do you support the establishment of a program to fund "high risk, high reward" research?

> The NIH includes a consideration of significance or reward along with the level of innovation in the review of all grant applications. Reviewers also consider the proposed approach and the feasibility of the project. Feasibility is frequently demonstrated by the inclusion of preliminary findings as a proof of concept. The development of the NIH Roadmap revealed the need to identify scientists with ideas that have the potential for high impact but which may be too underdeveloped to fare well in the traditional peer review process. In response, the NIH launched the NIH Director's Pioneer Award program aimed at supporting individuals with risk-taking, but ground breaking ideas ("high risk, high reward").

6. Do you think such projects should be subject to peer review?

> Peer reviewers are the key to identifying effective research projects in our traditional, project-focused review system, as well as in the process of identifying innovative scientists. For example, the NIH Director's Pioneer Award program uses a multi-level review process that facilitates the selection of individual scientists of exceptional creativity who propose pioneering approaches to major contemporary challenges in biomedical research.

7. Is there any reason to think that these projects cannot or should not be awarded competitively and transparently according to rules of grants and contracts?

> No. Peer review and effective grants management are necessary. We award grants for the best ideas and we ensure the proper conduct of and reporting on awarded projects.

You have been a strong advocate for NIH's system of peer review of grants and its independence from political pressures.

8. Do you believe the NIH Director should be able to de-fund a grant that has passed peer review by an institute?

> De-funding of peer-reviewed grants should only occur under extraordinary and appropriate circumstances. For example, in the case of financial or scientific fraud, or where patient safety is an issue. But in except in such circumstances, grants should not be defunded.

9. What potential dangers could result if an NIH Director began to pick and choose which grants to eliminate?

> As I have explained, grants should be defunded only under extraordinary and appropriate circumstances. For anyone to do otherwise would undermine NIH's long history of scientific objectivity and integrity.

10. What should be the NIH Director's role in assessing the agency's grant portfolio?

> Assessing the agency's grant portfolio should not be done by only one individual, whether the Director or someone else. But the NIH Director should ensure rigorous scientific assessment, using sound data and other unbiased evidence, and with the participation of experts and members of the public.

The National Research Council of the National Academy of Sciences recently recommended that appointments be made on the basis of their "scientific and technical knowledge and credentials and their professional and personal integrity."

11. Do you agree with this statement?

> Yes.

The National Research Council also stated that it is inappropriate to ask potential candidates for advisory committees about "nonrelevant information, such as voting record, political party affiliation, or position on particular policies."

12. Do you agree with this view?

> Yes.

Some have suggested that the NIH Director should prepare detailed reports and plans covering thousands of grants and hundreds of specific diseases.

13. What amount of reporting and what level of detail about grants is feasible?

> Feasible reporting is demonstrated by the various information resources and databases currently put out and maintained by the NIH. Such information includes broad overviews of general trends in biomedical research; amounts of NIH funding dedicated to specific diseases; award trends by State, institution and other parameters; descriptions of the research of every ongoing NIH grant; and the published results of all NIH-supported research. These resources are described below.
>
> Broad overviews, trends and highlights of NIH research can be found in the Director's annual early Spring testimony before Congress, which accompanies the annual budget request. More detail about specific research areas and programs can be found in the

annually published Budget Justification for NIH and the individual Budget Justifications for each NIH Institute and Center. All of this information can be found at the following URL http://officeofbudget.od.nih.gov/ui/HomePage.htm.

Estimates of funding for various diseases, conditions and research areas can be found at http://www.nih.gov/news/fundingresearchareas.htm which contains a table displaying funding levels based on actual grants, contracts, intramural research and other NIH support mechanisms. This information is updated annually. Actual amounts are reported for FY03 and FY04 and estimates are given for FY05 and FY06.

Award Trends can be found at the Office of Extramural Research site http://grants1.nih.gov/grants/award/awardtr.htm. This site contains a detailed breakdown of NIH funding by State, institution, research mechanism, responses to Requests for Applications and many other parameters.

Detailed descriptions of individual projects can be found using CRISP (Computer Retrieval of Information on Scientific Projects), which is a searchable biomedical database of federally-supported research conducted at universities, hospitals, and other research institutions (http://crisp.cit.nih.gov/).

Finally, all of the published results of NIH-supported grants and other mechanisms can be found using the searchable database PubMed. Furthermore, the new Public Access Policy, which was implemented by NIH on May 5, 2005 will create a stable archive, in PubMed Central, of peer-reviewed research publications resulting from NIH-funded research to ensure the permanent preservation of these vital published research findings. Complete information on the Public Access Policy can be found at http://www.nih.gov/about/publicaccess/.

14. What are the limits to the type of projections about future progress that an NIH Director can make?

NIH supports the discovery of scientific knowledge, knowing that the downstream impact of basic research on health is usually dependent on substantial further development of new knowledge by private industry, other public sector researchers, and economic factors. The full value of any given research finding may not be apparent at the time of discovery, and often reaches fruition after many years or in combination with other advances.

For example, a research effort to sequence a particular genome will, with relative certainty, accomplish its aim. In contrast, the discovery that a particular genetic pattern is associated with a disease process is significant scientific news, but it only suggests a direction for future research in the quest for an intervention. There is no certainty that this particular finding will lead to an intervention, and, even if it does, that outcome will depend on substantial further development of new knowledge and many other downstream events.

Progress from basic research to proof-of-concept to design and testing of an intervention is complex and nonlinear. The reasons for uncertainty associated with research are that:
- Outcomes are usually very difficult to foresee with any degree of accuracy.
- The full value of any given research finding is usually only barely visible at the time of discovery and reaches a state of fruition often after many years and in combination with other advances.
- The downstream impact of basic research usually is dependent on substantial further development of new knowledge by private industry, other public sector researchers, and economic factors.

Although research outcomes are challenging to predict, all NIH research is based on reaching goals. Moreover, in addition to findings related to the proposed hypothesis, outcomes may include unplanned results such as serendipitous discoveries and findings that narrow the avenue of the research focus (elimination discoveries), which can be just as significant.

In the context of the Government Performance and Results Act (GPRA), NIH presents a balanced portfolio of representative goals, ranging from low- to high-risk, and short- to long-term. NIH uses these performance-based goals with annual targets. The prospective target-based approach enhances the ability to predict and track progress; however, annual targets may need to be adjusted to incorporate new knowledge. These adjustments reflect the current state of the field and ensure the targets are meaningful to researchers, public, and NIH stakeholders. In addition, the qualitative performance reporting captures unplanned results that often prove significant in advancing the field. These adjustments may alter the initial projection, but ultimately enhance progress.

The draft legislation proposes to create a new division within the Office of the Director called the "Division of Program Coordination, Planning, and Strategic Initiatives" and would move several currently existing offices, including the Office of AIDS Research, the Office of Women's Health, and the Office of Rare Diseases, under the umbrella of the newly formed division.

15. Do you feel that you need a new division to manage these offices or will this merely create an unnecessary and redundant layer of bureaucracy?

   I believe that NIH requires a formal, institutionalized process led by the Division of Program Coordination, Planning, and Strategic Initiatives described in the draft legislation. I have already established a similar organization, the Office of Portfolio Analysis and Strategic Initiatives (OPASI) within the Office of the Director. The work of this office will not be unnecessary or redundant. OPASI will use a systematic approach to identify cross-cutting research and assess the entire NIH scientific portfolio.

16. Do you believe that it is possible for the Office of AIDS Research, for example, to operate under this Division of Program Coordination, Planning and Strategic Initiatives without losing any of its current authorities or changing any of its current functions? If not, what changes in OAR's current authorities and functions do you envision?

   I believe that program coordination offices can operate as part of the Division, as it is described in the draft legislation, or in conjunction with the Division should they not be incorporated into the Division, but should not and would not lose their statutory authorities or current functions.

APEX
TP_CF
9780150755064